MICHAEL MURPHY'S

BOOK OF DREAMS

Gill Books

Gill Books
Hume Avenue
Park West
Dublin 12
www.gillbooks.ie

Gill Books is an imprint of M.H. Gill & Co.

978 07171 7917 6

Design and print origination by O'K Graphic Design, Dublin
Copy-edited by Ellen Christie
Proofread by Esther Ní Dhonnacha
Printed by ScandBook AB, Sweden

This book is typeset in 11/17 pt Minion with headings in Lucida Calligraphy

The paper used in this book comes from the wood pulp of managed forests. For every tree felled, at least one tree is planted, thereby renewing natural resources.

A CIP catalogue record for this book is available from the British Library.

5 4 3 2

*For all dreamers everywhere, that the poetry of dreams
may enrich the prose of your everyday.*

About the Author

*M*ichael Murphy is a broadcaster, psychoanalyst, author and lecturer. He has worked in RTÉ as a newscaster and award-winning television producer/director, and is well known from his interviews on radio and television.

Michael is a Registered Practitioner member of the Association for Psychoanalysis and Psychotherapy in Ireland. He works full time as a French-trained Psychoanalyst at his practice in Sandyford, Dublin, where he is the Director of Psychological Therapy Services.

Michael lectures in Communications at the Park Studio and the Milltown Institute in Dublin, and works as a Communications Consultant with the T-Space Organisation, primarily for Irish governmental organisations.

In 2009, Michael published a number one bestselling literary memoir, *At Five in the Afternoon*, dealing with his battle with prostate cancer. A sequel, *The House of Pure Being*, was published in autumn 2013 and reached the top ten. A poetry collection, *The Republic of Love*, was published in summer 2013 and was the first poetry book to enter the top ten list in Ireland since Seamus Heaney won the Nobel Prize. Michael's second collection of poetry, *A Chaplet of Roses*, was published in autumn 2016. The *Irish Independent* has described him as 'an author of importance'.

Michael was awarded an honorary degree by the National University of Ireland, Galway. The citation reads, 'Through his outstanding work as a broadcaster, psychoanalyst and writer, Michael Murphy has made an important and valuable contribution to Irish society and beyond ...'

Contents

Foreword

We have all come to know Michael Murphy through his work as a broadcaster, producer and television personality. Michael's voice permeated our homes with an air of sincere urgency and care when he broadcast the news on radio or television. His was the voice you listened to, not just because of what he was saying, but because of how he was saying it. Michael expressed himself with such articulate care and compassion that we felt somehow better about ourselves: it made us feel that we were worthy of such care.

Michael has devoted himself to careful, artful articulation as a broadcaster, writer and psychoanalyst. This was evident in his first book, *At Five in the Afternoon*, in which he documented his struggle with prostate cancer and invited us to witness his courageous journey. Following this he passionately explored sexuality, complex human relationships and commitment in his second prose work, *The House of Pure Being*. Michael's passion and engagement with the human condition continued when he published two collections of poetry, *The Republic of Love* and *A Chaplet of Roses*, in which he took us on an emotional tour that left us reflecting on, sharing and celebrating life.

This present work of Michael's once again challenges us. This time it is a challenge to explore the unconscious through our dreams. The book is a natural progression in Michael's writing, and it shows itself to be a thoughtful integration of his years of psychoanalytic practice, nuanced communication skills, curiosity and abundant humanity. Armed with these years of analytic experience and a profound knowledge of psychoanalytic theory informed by the writings of Jung, Freud, Lacan and others, Michael respectfully and warmly analyses the dreamscape.

In *Michael Murphy's Book of Dreams*, Michael has intelligently and artfully provided interpretations and hypotheses that are free from psychoanalytic jargon, yet not lacking in depth. He maintains the sanctity of the original dream, and respectfully offers insights to decode the prompts from the unconscious that provide direction and support to the dreamer. Michael conducts his analyses with warmth, compassion and an instinct for the fulcrum message of the dream.

His attention to detail is reflected in his painstaking delving into the possible meanings of words through etymology and ambiguity, where he examines the symbolism of dreams from all perspectives.

Michael opens with a succinct yet thorough introduction to the basic functions of the dream, and he introduces the process of analysis in an understandable, friendly manner, which illustrates how the unconscious communicates through the dream drama.

Following his introduction, Michael documents brief dreamscapes which he analyses. This is a characteristically brave departure, as Michael has only the dream upon which to work: he has no knowledge of the dreamers nor of their lives. However, undeterred, he arrives at deep and potentially significant therapeutic findings for those whose dreams he analyses.

Michael's work also challenges the professional psychotherapist, and encourages them to invest time and effort in understanding their client's unconscious communications and dreams. While *Michael Murphy's Book of Dreams* is not a dream interpretation manual, it offers the professional reader a courageous illustration of this work in action that cannot but inspire them.

Michael's approach is respectful, curious and informed. He is at times serious and considered, and at other times, he incarnates the humorous trickster, encouraging his clients to view themselves with compassion and humour. Michael's approach is always respectful and supportive, which ensures his clients' safety.

The dreams are characteristically oblique and obscure when examined literally, and their meanings are hard to discern initially. Michael's transparent and thorough examination of each dream helps the reader see the dream from the analyst's perspective, and witness companionably the process of analysis.

This collection of contemporary Irish dreams will further our insight into the Irish psyche and how we make sense of our conscious and unconscious processes. Michael's work will doubtless continue to contribute to our understanding and acceptance of ourselves into the future. I am delighted to witness this work. Michael has yet again given us a courageous and compassionate look at our humanity by illuminating our unconscious processes, and showing how their integration into our consciousness can enrich and bring balance into our daily lives.

Dr Patrick Randall
Consultant Clinical & Forensic Psychologist
Director, Forensic Psychological Services, Dún Laoghaire, Co. Dublin

Introduction

*E*veryone dreams, but not everyone remembers their dreams, which is a pity. Because by paying attention to our dreams, we can ground ourselves in the deepest truth of our being, and make wiser choices that work towards our greater good. Consciously, we see our lives as if through the tiny viewfinder on a mobile phone, whereas unconsciously, we see our lives as if writ large on a massive cinemascope screen. So it's sensible to allow this bigger picture – as seen in our dreams – to inform our lives, and to follow our dreams.

Dreams have played an important role in many cultures throughout history. In the ancient world, dreams were seen as messages from the gods. The biblical patriarchs Abraham and Jacob were guided by their dreams, and so too was Joseph in the New Testament. The Egyptian god of dreams, Serapis, had many temples throughout Egypt. In Greek religion, Morpheus was worshipped as the god of dreams. He formed the images and visions that communicated what the gods wanted the dreamer to know. Visits were made to the temples of Asclepius, the god of medicine, for healing guidance from dreams. This ancient wisdom of dreams, which has been revered over thousands of years, is available to us today when we honour our dreams.

Dreams arise from bursts of activity in a biologically ancient part of the mid brain. The limbic system has to do with emotions and plays a role in memory storage. It also includes the most primitive, instinctive part of the brain, responsible for REM sleep. REM or dream sleep evolved 130 million years ago. Dreams occur regularly throughout the night every 90 minutes, each episode persisting from 5 to 40 minutes. They account for a quarter of each night's sleep. The presence of REM sleep in many species, such as dogs, cats, horses, elephants, probably all higher animals, is shown by the movements and sounds they make while dreaming, which indicates that dreams must perform a crucial survival function in mammals.

Scientific research shows that dreams are involved with memory storage. Dreams are a neural process whereby information essential to the survival of the species gathered during the day is reprocessed into memory during REM sleep, so that our collective survival strategies are updated. Our own private dreams also contribute to this collective tapestry. By paying attention to our dreams, we can draw on this vital, unconscious resource to more appropriately react to the circumstances we face, and to make better choices that will contribute to our future survival and success.

Dreams are formulated in a pictorial language that we can only understand when we put the images into words. That's why it is a good idea to keep a dream journal in which to write down our dreams. However, it is wise to discuss our dreams only with people we love or who support us, because our dreams are very revealing self-portrayals. They reveal certain situations in our unconscious in symbolic form. The words we use when describing them are sacred, as they arise from our soul. Far from being ephemeral, dreams are a basic fact of experience, and they should be honoured as such. Often we can also experience the emotion carried by a dream at night while we sleep, and this can carry over into the next day while we are awake. We can then better understand the dream's symbolic significance by analysing those feelings, no matter how uncomfortable, unsettling or even consoling they might be.

Dreams chart a hero's journey through life, rather like a film. We are the producer and the director, we choose the camera angles, we write the drama, and we commission the actors. The archetypal hero pattern in dreams shows the process or the various rites of passage that we need to undergo in order to accomplish our psychological growth. This journey goes from childhood through the adolescent transition into early maturity, followed by the midlife transition into middle age and the late-life transition into late maturity and old age. This life journey leads us to become more mature human beings.

There are many different elements and themes that occur regularly in dreams, which act as signposts that mark the stages in our spiritual journey. Identifying these can help us to decipher the metaphorical and figurative nature of dreams, so that we may understand and be guided towards maturity by what they communicate.

The Animus is the masculine side of a woman's unconscious. There are four stages of this symbolic inner development for a woman that often manifest in dreams. First, an Animus figure may appear as a male figure who personifies physical power, such as an athletic champion. This is followed by an action hero, a man who takes initiatives in the world. Third is a more intellectual figure, such as a professor or a philosopher. Finally, the fourth inner male figure in a woman's dreams essentially incarnates meaning and purpose for her. He is a well-rounded figure, who incorporates all of the three previous transformations, and can be regarded as a wise, old man.

The Anima is the feminine side of a man's unconscious. The first stage in the development of the Anima or inner feminine is often personified in dreams as a woman who represents instinct and sexual relations. The second is more a romantic figure, but one who is still characterised by sexual elements. The third stage corresponds to the goddess or the Virgin Mary, which is a symbol of love raised to the heights of spiritual devotion. The final and fourth stage is a figure who yields wisdom, and can be represented by the personification of wisdom known as Sophia, who was the central concept of Hellenistic religion, corresponding to the Holy Spirit in Christianity.

The goal in paying conscious attention to this unconscious evolution in our psyches is to bring more balance into our lives, and ultimately to become wise and whole human beings. The Animus and Anima archetypes, which have the characteristics of the opposite gender, are a guide for our inner world and are personified in Animus or Anima figures in dreams. These figures have many gifts to share with us from the unconscious masculine or feminine within, not least in sexual matters, but also in broadening and balancing out our personalities.

Shadow dreams feature people of the same sex as the dreamer. A Shadow figure often appears as inferior or negative, and embodies the unpleasant qualities in ourselves that we prefer to hide. For example, a Shadow figure may appear in a man's dream as a man trying to break into his house. The intruder may embody qualities the dreamer was forced to repress by parents or teachers when he was young. However, these qualities – like being streetwise, confrontational, stubborn or belligerent – could help him now as an adult if he were to bring them back into use.

There's always a secret sympathy with this rejected part of our personality that reveals itself in our dreams. We like to help the enemy within, which shows up in the embarrassing mistakes that we make or in our slips of the tongue. If we remained in blissful ignorance of the repressed negative qualities in our Shadow, we would be in danger of being possessed by them and of acting them out. Our dreams can alert us in time to this danger. We can also project these negative attitudes outwards and wrongly scapegoat others, since often we don't recognise these traits as our own until a dream points them out.

Many dreams concern the Self, the archetype of wholeness and the unifying centre of the psyche. The Self is usually perceived in dreams as other, for example, as God, the sun, the president, the queen, or even as language or speech that comes from a numinous other place. Such dreams induce awe.

Helpful animals can appear in dreams to assist the hero in completing his tasks. We can ask why a dream shows a crafty fox, as opposed to a far-seeing eagle, or a powerful Rottweiler. It is because animals are closer to their instincts than most people, and they remind us in an era of smartphones and laptops that we, too, need to use our instinctive animal know-how. Shakespeare, who empathically understood human nature, and whose brilliant mind could describe our qualities in zoomorphic terms, listed 'hog in sloth, fox in stealth, wolf in greediness, dog in madness, lion in prey' (*King Lear*). All of these animals appear in our dreams and carry those references to this day. For example, a snake may appear in dreams when the mind is deviating from its instinctual basis and needs to get back on track with territorial behaviour, defence or competitive striving.

Dreams often present Persona problems. The Persona is the way we appear to others, the face we put on. This can be illustrated in dreams through the clothes we wear or don't wear. These dreams can tell us that we over-identify with the professional role we play, and need to shed that, or that an unbalanced Persona is causing us unnecessary stress.

Trickster and Shapeshifter figures appear in our dreams when we take matters too seriously. Clown figures or the Shakespearean fool, for example, challenge and set new limits for us, astonish us and awaken us to different perspectives and new ways of approaching difficulties.

It can be useful to summarise your dream in a sentence: 'I had a dream last night that I killed somone' or 'I dreamt that my teeth fell out'. Dreams of dying or killing someone concern the death of the attitudes that the victims embody, or worn-out ways of approaching life that we need to shed. Teeth dreams have to do with times of transition – getting older when once upon a time a person's teeth fell out as we aged (with the potential to regress to childhood). The appearance of teeth in dreams also suggests we should get outside help with our problem (we don't take out our own teeth; we seek the help of dentists). Wedding dreams represent the coming together of the opposites in our personalities, often giving birth to an unexpected third position that partakes of the two alternatives. The goal of wholeness is to be able to move between these two opposing sides comfortably. And a wedding in dreams also demonstrates to us that a transformation is possible, which is consoling. Doing the Leaving Cert and not being prepared for it shows that a transition is occurring: there's a new challenge facing us in our lives, and we need to get up to speed with this examination, and wake up to the situation in order to prepare for it properly.

Finally, a nightmare is a dream that shouts at us to pay attention to a potential danger. It mobilises our fight or flight responses.

Dreams reveal our unconscious mind. By paying attention to our dreams and trying to decipher them, we can get additional data upon which to base our conscious choices so that we are more in tune with our true selves, which embrace both the unconscious and consciousness. Dreams always relate us to the age-old concerns of humanity: feeding, fighting, fleeing and fornication. By owning our dreams and playing around with what they have to say, by looking at the dream from as many perspectives as possible since everything and everybody in the dream refers to us, we can increase the influence of their creative power in our lives.

The dreams in this collection are contemporary and reflect Ireland today. They were chosen because they are commonly occurring, and show themes and motifs that can apply to any individual. The dreams were written down as they were related, and so reflect the dreamers' sometimes unusual use of language. They came to me from a wide variety of public and private sources to analyse in my work as a psychoanalyst.

When I work with a client's dream in the privacy of the consulting room, their personal associations to the dream have pride of place, in order to allow the individual truth of their personalities have its say as much as possible. Apart from giving the sex of the dreamer, the dreams in this volume are seldom amplified by many subjective associations, which serves to protect the client. The names of the dreamers have also been changed to ensure their privacy. On the one hand, the lack of context and subjective detail is a loss. On the other hand, it's also an opportunity that allows the objective structure of these dreams to be analysed in a way that demonstrates how any dream can be analysed.

I hope that this book of dreams will help others to both analyse and live out the wisdom of their own dreams. Thus even in today's sceptical world, which largely ignores the sacred and has forgotten the underlying myths which support our civilisation, dreams can continue to be considered as messages from the gods within!

1

Anima and Animus Dreams

*T*he unconscious side of our personality is represented in dreams by a person of the opposite sex. The feminine side of a man's unconscious is known as the Anima, while the masculine side of a woman's unconscious is called the Animus. Both the Anima and Animus represent a person's soul, and their personification as Anima and Animus figures in a dream can lead us to make a connection with our unconscious side, which compensates for deficiencies in our conscious attitudes.

The character of a man's femininity and a woman's masculinity are formed by our mothers and fathers, who were influenced in turn by their parents, and so on. The Anima and Animus figures in our dreams, which derive from our ancestry, accompany us on our inner journey, and lead us towards discovering our individual meaning. For example, we often choose to fall in love with people who embody this projection of our ancient, ancestral soul, because at some deep level we realise that they are compatible with us and balance out our personalities. Therefore the Anima and Animus are responsible for finding the right marriage partner! However, at a later stage in the development of our relationships, perhaps seven or eight years into a marriage, this projection of the embodiment of our Anima or Animus onto our partner has to be withdrawn and recognised for what it is: an eternal potential within, which properly belongs to ourselves. True love can then deepen the relationship. However, if this soul image is not properly understood and integrated back into the personality, the disappointment it engenders can split the relationship apart.

Anima and Animus manifest in both negative and positive forms as an inner power. A positive Anima in a man is life-giving, spontaneous, creative and inspiring; it carries the emotional side of his nature. The Anima allows a man to be receptive to the irrational, to have a capacity for personal love, a feeling for nature, and the ability to relate to the unconscious. The Anima compensates for man's logical mind. What's more, in our dreams the Anima figure puts a man in tune with the inner values that are correct for him, and opens him up to profound inner depths, guiding him and mediating his inner world. In tune with his Anima figure, he is able to incarnate this experience of the feminine within through writing, painting, sculpture, musical composition or dance. Negative aspects of the Anima can show up when a man is moody or touchy, irritable, rigid, pedantic, depressed, uncertain or insecure; when he is behaving like the negative stereotype of a woman, prone to waspish, poisonous or effeminate remarks.

In a woman, negative aspects of the Animus can surface in being stridently angry, argumentative, controlling or obstinate with absolute convictions; again, like the negative stereotype of a man. Negative Animus qualities also manifest as coldness and complete inaccessibility; as brutality, recklessness and malevolent silence. One can rarely contradict a sweeping Animus opinion because in the most general way it's usually correct, although anyone being so adamant is never warranted. The negative Animus figure also personifies dreamy thoughts full of desire and judgements about how things ought to be but aren't. These things can serve to cut off a woman from the reality of life. On the other hand, positive aspects to the Animus drive a woman to get things done and be focused, always leading towards positive and healthy life-giving relationships with other people. A positive Animus gives a woman spiritual firmness and compensates for her softer, maternal qualities. He opens her to new, creative ideas. Often the Animus takes form in dreams as a group of men, symbolising the received wisdom of the collective, rather than being solely an individual contribution.

Barry's dream of the crying girl

✦ ✧ ✦ ✧ ✦

I had a dream I walked into a room and found a crying girl. I looked away and when I looked back, she was drowning in a river. – Barry

✦ ✧ ✦ ✧ ✦

This is a dream about an Anima figure, a representative of the feminine side of the male soul. Barry's Anima presents as a girl. A female child originally had the meaning of a maidservant. So the girl is presented to Barry as a servant – one who serves another for wages – she is not Barry's equal, nor is she a grown-up, mature woman. Indeed the history of the word 'girl' refers to a young person of either sex, so this Anima figure is quite undifferentiated, and is perhaps even a male suffering from connotations of prissiness, oversensitivity and effeminacy. So we can conclude that Barry is having a dream about a negative Anima figure.

According to the drama of the dream, Barry ignores what he should notice: when he sees the distress of the Anima who is crying, he looks away, instead of being protective and moving towards her to comfort her and find out what's wrong. This scene serves to underline Barry's gauche immaturity being expressed in the dream. Then in a moment of increased tension, when Barry looks back, the girl is drowning in a river. Drowning, or dying by submersion in water, is a metaphor that describes the crying girl's feelings of helplessness, and symbolises her grief and sadness at the situation. Shakespeare used the same motif in his play *Hamlet*, when Ophelia drowns in a river.

This is a warning dream. Barry is shown in the most graphic terms that he is in danger of losing his feminine side, which has to do with relating to others and employing his softer feelings, and which has personified in his dream as an undeveloped girl. His Anima is in danger of death by drowning, be it through her tears or the river.

The dream presents this situation to Barry without showing its conclusion, so there is still time to try to save her. The dream gives Barry a choice: to do nothing, or to rescue the representative of his soul before it's too late.

This is a good example of why we should pay attention to what the unconscious shows us in dreams. If Barry doesn't act on the dream, his Anima figure may not have the opportunity to grow up and become his equal.

Barry uses the word 'drowning'. We often use that word figuratively to indicate being overwhelmed, inundated, flooded or submerged. So we can ask the question: what is causing Barry's inner feminine side to drown? Is there a grief or sorrow in his life that is so overwhelming he's unable to face up to it in a mature way? Does this grief come from his childhood, when something had such a traumatic effect that it left him emotionally frozen? What is blunting Barry's finer feelings, coarsening him, leaving him in danger of being swallowed up? Could it be drink, for example, because the base of the Old English verb 'to drown' also means 'to drink'?

Barry will be able to recognise what catastrophe is underway in his life that has left his Anima figure in such an undeveloped state that she's in danger of death. The good news is that he's being given a chance to do something about it; to bring his Anima back to life through employing the gifts that his inner female can offer him by way of service, and by incarnating her more mature qualities in his everyday life.

Conor's dream of the woman in black

✦ ✧ ✦ ✧ ✦

I occasionally dream that I open the curtains and there's a woman standing across the road. She's dressed in black and staring at me, and it's night. – Conor

✦ ✧ ✦ ✧ ✦

*T*his dream, which Conor says he has now and then, is about the 'gaze' or the 'look'. The characteristic of the gaze or the look is that we have to read into it. We can make a guess at what it means, but we don't know what it is about until the other person tells us. This sense of someone staring at us induces anxiety because we lose autonomy by knowing we're a visible object for another person's unreadable gaze. In Irish society it is not considered polite to stare, and that training goes back to our childhood and the prohibitions that came from our parents. So a taboo is being broken here.

The existentialist philosopher Jean-Paul Sartre pointed out that when a person is surprised by the gaze of the other, he is reduced to shame. Conor says, 'I open the curtains and there's a woman … staring at me'. The woman's look reduces Conor to feeling shamed and objectified.

The fact that he opens the curtains means that he, too, is looking. In the theatre of this dream Conor dramatically stages the male gaze, from which we see things from the perspective of a heterosexual man. The act of the curtains opening is constructed for the pleasure of this male viewer, which is deeply rooted in patriarchal ideologies.

Presumably Conor is looking through the glass of a window, which means that he's cut off from relating directly with the woman – cut off from feeling. The woman is also 'standing across the road', so in the dream the reciprocity of this objectifying distance from both the male and the female is doubly emphasized.

When Conor looks, the woman in black is already staring back at him, but from a point at which he's unable to do the seeing – Conor can say nothing more about what the female sees, because the dream dramatises Conor as having only the one, narrow masculine perspective, whereas it could have incorporated both angles. So the dream also points to the alienating split in our subjectivity that we're sometimes made aware of, and which is expressed in Conor's dream through the field of vision.

The woman in black is an Anima figure, which means she's representing Conor's inner feminine. It looks as if Conor is seriously split off from that side of his personality – alienated from it – which is probably why he's having this dream. The drama of the dream, in which the action is represented by a silent and motionless *tableau vivant*, shows Conor that he needs to open himself up to relate to the Anima figure, person to person, in order to experience intimacy, and not just view her from 'across the road', or through the narrow lens of male attitudes. He needs to understand that women may be 'other', but they are not alien! Maybe Conor is viewing too much porn on his computer screen instead of relating to a flesh-and-blood woman. The fixed gaze of a woman dressed in black and staring has roots in being solid, rigid or stiff, which carry sexual overtones as well as having the quality of being immobile.

The woman in Conor's dream is dressed in black, and the scene takes place in the black of night as well. What could that mean? The staring woman could be in mourning or feeling depressed, dressed corporately as a lawyer or for business, or she could be wearing a little black dress for a night out: all of these possibilities are contained within the dream.

Her black dress could also represent an unconscious part of Conor's personality that has not been lived out yet, known as the Shadow. The Shadow is made up of qualities that the dreamer deems incompatible with his image. It has connotations of being dark, shady, unsubstantial and fleeting, and has figurative and applied meanings such as being ghost-like, being an imperfect representation, or even moral darkness. The Shadow normally appears in dreams as a figure of the same sex as the dreamer, but it can also contaminate the Anima with its darkness. Therefore the 'night' atmosphere of this dream could be dramatising the presence of the Shadow, which suggests Conor is in need of the light of consciousness.

Conor is being asked to engage with this dream, and to make conscious efforts to connect with the undeveloped feminine in him. Perhaps he can do this through embracing his vulnerability, even if it's still at an immature stage. But he should also try to connect in a real way with members of the opposite sex that he comes into contact with in his daily life, and to remove the barriers highlighted in his dream that block him off from his most intimate feelings. If he does this, the dream will gradually stop occuring, only repeating occasionally until he properly understands and acts upon what it is bringing to his attention.

Anne's dream of her dead cousin

✦ ✧ ✦ ✧ ✦

I always have the same dream. It's about my cousin who died 10 years ago. I dream that we're in the kitchen having tea and he asks me why I won't talk to him. I've been having panic attacks over this dream because it is scary. Does it mean anything? – Anne

✦ ✧ ✦ ✧ ✦

There's no need to have panic attacks over this dream, or indeed any dream. A person's unconscious has their best interests at heart, working for their health and happiness, so this dream occurs repeatedly for a positive reason. The dream returns in the same form because it brings to Anne's attention what hasn't been heard by her or fully understood. The panic attacks and scary feelings that the dream induces are designed to get Anne to do something about the situation.

This is an Animus dream in which Anne's cousin is a personification of her unconscious masculine side. In addition, he's a blood relative, so physically shares the same gene pool as her. This underlines that he's very much a part of her, and is a positive expression of her soul.

Anne describes the scene as 'in the kitchen having tea', which is a very normal, relaxed and companionable situation, taking place in the informal heart of the house where we would feel perfectly at home with a member of our family. This intimate activity shows that there's no threat, because we wouldn't have tea with somebody who wishes us harm, and Anne gives no indication of that being the case.

There are just two pieces of descriptive information that Anne shares about her cousin, her positive Animus figure. The first is that he died 10 years ago. So Anne is having tea with an Animus figure who has been dead for 10 years. The dream could have chosen a living man to portray this situation, but instead the dream states clearly that Anne's Animus figure is dead, or at least is 10 years past its sell-by date! So we need to ask what masculine attitudes Anne is holding onto that are out of date.

There's also an ambiguity here because this Animus figure is alive in the private informal space of her kitchen, where Anne can be herself and which traditionally was regarded as the domain of the female. A kitchen is also a place of transformation, where food is changed from its raw state into nourishing meals, to be generously shared with intimates. So this setting also carries the potential for transformation in Anne's life.

The second piece of information is that while they're having tea, her cousin asks her why she won't talk to him. There are a number of things we can say about such a question, and about the type of person who asks it. For a start, by asking what has gone wrong in the relationship between them, he is making a very direct and unambiguous challenge, which requires a degree of courage. It's also possible that the person who asks such a question might feel victimised in some way, or perhaps is hurt because of Anne's behaviour. The question expresses a judgement and a reproach, in which Anne is blamed by her cousin for her refusal to talk to him. In the question, 'Why won't you talk to me?', the verb 'won't' – meaning 'will not', indicating intention and volition – is a very strong verb of refusal, more usually employed by a young child, who doesn't have the polite, nuanced vocabulary of an adult. The question is also an appeal: 'Why won't you talk to me?' Anne's Animus figure is issuing an invitation to her to reply and to engage in a truthful dialogue with him, while also offering the possibility to heal what's amiss. All of which sounds very positive indeed.

Yet Anne's reaction isn't in accord with the clear invitation to speak. Her Animus figure has initiated a dialogue with her in this dream in order to demonstrate that Anne has a stubborness to her character that's immovable and unyielding: she won't talk. Perhaps it's a childish reaction. But by putting words to how she's feeling, and by taking the first step of being open and receptive to her dream instead of having panic attacks, Anne will not only be able to express herself, but will be able to affirm her place in the world.

She says, 'I've been having panic attacks over this dream because it is scary.' I presume Anne thinks the dream is scary because a dead person visits her in her sleep, but this misses the point of what the drama of the dream is trying to convey. Anne is suffering from unreasoning fear because she won't put herself into speech, which would have the effect of defining who she is, and thereby relieve the build-up of emotional stress. Her panic attacks and scary feelings have been transposed from the dream onto the idea of death. She asks, 'Does it mean anything?' So, again on the death theme, maybe Anne is really asking whether the visitation by her dead cousin is really to announce her own death.

The dream is asking Anne to start a dialogue with the qualities that her male cousin embodied. If she engages with those qualities and begins to use them in her own life, then the nightmare quality of this dream will cease. Now, it could be that her cousin wasn't a nice person, in which case she should look at this dream head on, and make up her mind about the male qualities he embodied. But by engaging with the dream in a constructive way, she will put it – and her cousin – to rest. If, as the dream seems to suggest, she can have a conversation with this cousin in the relaxed and transformative atmosphere of her kitchen, then she should do that as soon as she can. She should have a dialogue with him in her mind, thinking of the subjects of conversation she used to have with him, and tackle anything that hasn't been dealt with and that's still outstanding in the their relationship, which was severed too soon by death. Above all, Anne should talk, put everything into words and not bottle it up!

Aidan's dream of Paloma Faith

✦ ✧ ✦ ✧ ✦

I dreamt last night that I got it on big time with the singer Paloma Faith. It's weird because I don't find her that attractive at all. It was fantastic though! – Aidan

✦ ✧ ✦ ✧ ✦

*P*aloma Faith is an Anima figure for Aidan, the representative of his inner feminine. He has projected his unconscious female qualities outwards onto Paloma Faith, and what positive qualities they are.

Paloma Faith is a very accomplished woman in her thirties of both northern European and Latin heritage. She is a singer/songwriter and actress who is heavily influenced by soul and jazz, and known for her retro style. She's a bright and determined woman, which shows that Aidan is having a dream about a positive Anima figure.

Interestingly, Paloma is a singer, which is a wonderfully creative expression of the human soul. Singing is pure feeling, and a singer puts her whole being into her voice, thereby reaching out and moving other people with her singing.

In his dream, Aidan says that he 'got it on big time' with the singer, which is a euphemism for having sex. And sex is one of the most intimate connections we can make with another human being. As well as enjoying sex, Aidan is getting in touch 'big time' with his creative feminine side, which is a spontaneous movement towards life – to the earth, to emotions, towards people and things. This connection will encourage Aidan to become more involved with the community, and it will balance out his one-sided, consciously masculine perspective, which his dream suggests is too narrow.

Aidan points out that getting it on with Paloma is 'weird', which is a revealing word choice. Presumably he used the word in the sense of 'odd' – which is a recent meaning, first used by the poet Shelley in 1815 – but for over a thousand years, the word 'weird' meant the ability to control the fate of men. Even in Middle English it referred to the three 'Fates' or goddesses who controlled human destiny, like the three 'Weird Sisters' in Shakespeare's play *Macbeth*. So unconsciously in his use of that word, Aidan recognises the power that his inner goddess has over him.

Indicating his ambivalence, Aidan says, 'I don't find her that attractive at all'. The original meaning of the word 'attractive' referred to the ability to draw out diseased matter as a means of treatment, and to ingest nutriment, which points to the healing qualities of his Anima figure. On a conscious level, by saying he doesn't find her that attractive, he's also misreading his feminine qualities, which seem to be stuck at that first stage in the development of the Anima: instinct and sexual relations. Possibly Aidan is being too 'blokey' by lacking feeling and empathy, which, interestingly, are the very qualities being offered by his Anima figure. He should be more accepting of these gifts of feeling and empathy being offered by his inner Paloma before he continues with the dating game, so that he'll be better able to find a suitable soulmate and life-partner. Although I appreciate Aidan may just be starting out on that particular journey, and may need to play the field first.

We can see that Aidan recognises the need to fully embrace his feminine side through his positive conclusion about the dream: 'It was fantastic though!' The word 'fantastic' derives from the Greek '*phantázein*' meaning to make visible or to have visions, which are seen in the imagination and in dreaming, or experienced as a supernatural occurrence.

Finally, Paloma is the Spanish word for 'dove', the symbol of peace, and the name can also be understood in Christian tradition as referring to the Holy Spirit. Faith comes from the Latin, meaning trust or belief, especially religious belief. In this sense, we can understand the visionary dream as the Anima figure leading a man to get in touch with his spiritual side. According to this dream, Aidan has the potential to reach the third goddess phase in his psychological development, which has incorporated instinctive, sexual elements. All that is left is to learn is the wisdom of this wonderful dream!

Darragh's dream of being with a girl he had never seen before

✦ ✧ ✦ ✧ ✦

I was at a party and was with a girl I had never seen before. Out of nowhere my girlfriend showed up. She sat on her own and everyone started shouting at her. She got really upset, but I ended up leaving with the girl I had never seen before. – Darragh

✦ ✧ ✦ ✧ ✦

*T*he Anima figure is the representative of a man's soul, leading him to get in contact with his feminine side. But in Darragh's dream, the Anima is split between two figures: a girl he's never seen before, on the one hand, and his girlfriend who showed up 'out of nowhere', on the other hand. This displays two aspects of the feminine, and also dramatises a conflict. In the concluding act of the dream, Darragh ends up leaving with the girl he had never seen before.

It is important that Darragh takes this dream seriously. The dream draws to his attention the fact that there are aspects to the feminine that he has never seen before, which are different to those displayed by his girlfriend. So as a starting point, it might be useful to compare and contrast the qualities of the girl in the dream and his girlfriend's attributes.

He says that when his girlfriend shows up, 'everyone started shouting at her', which suggests that he's angry with his girlfriend for cramping his style at playing away, because the 'everyone' in the dream is really an expression of some aspect of his personality. His girlfriend 'sat on her own' presumably to make the obvious point that she's being two-timed and 'got really upset'. This shows that Darragh anticipates her reaction to his discovery of new aspects of the feminine that he's never seen before: he feels that his girlfriend won't like it, and she'll cause a scene.

Now, the word 'upset' is an interesting one. It originally meant to set up or erect, and only turned into its opposite meaning in the early 1800s: to overturn and feel distressed. Both usages are implied here. And this duality also extends into the dramatic action of the dream. It could well be that the girl he had never seen before could also represent an aspect of his girlfriend that is waiting to be discovered through Darragh making a commitment to an ongoing loving relationship with her.

Finally, it's important to state that this exploration of the feminine is more an internal journey for Darragh rather than a projection of his feelings outwards onto other women. The dream asks him to put his own house in order first, to examine his unconscious desires as expressed in his dream, and then consciously live them out in an ethically responsible manner, so that neither he nor others end up getting hurt. If his girlfriend holds 90 per cent of his inner Anima figure, then he'll be compatible with her. If, on the other hand, she only embodies, say, 60 per cent, that means that there's 40 per cent of his inner feminine that is stray and ungrounded. Then the reality is there might be an ongoing problem with commitment for him going forward. So it's time for Darragh to face up to these choices and to make some thoughtful decisions about his life!

2

Shadow Dreams

*T*he Shadow appears in dreams as a person of the same sex. The Shadow usually contains values that are needed by our consciousness, but that exist in a form difficult for us to integrate because we regard them as liabilities. When we become aware of the Shadow, the values it embodies are often imbued with feelings of guilt, and we feel that we'll be rejected by others and horribly exposed if they come to light.

The Shadow contains the hidden, repressed and unfavourable aspects of our personality. At its core is a potential for pure evil, which we all could be capable of bringing forth given the right circumstances.

The Shadow also contains good qualities, normal instincts and creative impulses that we have jettisoned. The need we felt once upon a time to adapt to the expectations of our parents, teachers and society in the course of growing up meant that the energy in qualities that were perceived as undesirable, or indeed reprehensible, was removed from view and fell into the Shadow.

These 'bold' qualities need to be rescued and brought back into use so that we can fire on all cylinders and draw energy from our seven deadly sins as well as from our seven cardinal virtues. We keep pushing our virtues to the front in the vain hope of disguising or being rid of our vices. However, we can't be rid of them, so we should stop trying to keep them quiet. We need to let them have their say in as positive a manner as possible. The bold qualities that are now silent and dormant have to be mined for their energy and integrated into our personality as best we can.

To own our Shadow is a painful and potentially terrifying experience, so much so that we usually deny the existence of our Shadow and, instead, project it outwards onto other people. This is done unconsciously as an act of ego-preservation. This act of unconscious cunning explains the ancient practice of 'scapegoating'. It underlies all kinds of prejudices against others, for example: the enemy; the treacherous stranger who's taking our jobs; those who have a different approach to sexual matters, politics or religion; or the evil intruder to our dreams who's trying to break into our house, the place where we live. Paradoxically, these 'intruders' could be bringing the gift of qualities that we could benefit from.

The Shadow represents the opposite side of our civilised ego, and embodies the qualities one dislikes most in other people. It represents unknown or little-known attributes and qualities that perhaps a person denies in himself but can clearly see in other people – selfishness, laziness, unreal fantasies and schemes, carelessness, addictions, different sexualities or an inordinate love of money. All of these projections are in fact a personification of part of ourselves we don't recognise, or don't want to recognise so we project it onto others. We don't want to welcome the enemy home as our brother.

The Shadow also has a protective function. It is the Shadow that makes us wary of the enemy or the stranger, which is a survival function causing us to not trust anything strange that could be predatory or hostile.

A person becomes enlightened and wise by bringing the darkness in the Shadow to our consciousness; by recognising our prejudices. This is a disagreeable process and therefore not very popular. The Shadow is like another human being with whom one has to get along – sometimes by giving in, sometimes by resisting, and more often by loving – because at some level the rejected Shadow is hurting. It only becomes hostile when it is ignored or misunderstood. And because the core of the Shadow is evil, it is extremely dangerous to deny the existence of our Shadow, because then we're at greater risk of being taken over by it, with disastrously destructive results.

Since the Shadow is a part of ourselves, we support it unconsciously, which can be seen in our impulsive actions, or in Freudian slips of the tongue that trick us into telling the truth despite our protestations to the contrary.

Albert's dream of Roy Keane helping him move house

✦ ✧ ✦ ✧ ✦

Last night I dreamt that I was best friends with Roy Keane. He was helping me move house and was driving my stuff in a van. No matter how much we loaded the van, the flat never emptied. – Albert

✦ ✧ ✦ ✧ ✦

*R*oy Keane comes up in this dream as Albert's best friend, with all the implications of loyalty and intimacy that such a relationship implies. And there's a big move underway in Albert's personality, as described by this metaphorical drama. In the picture painted by Albert's dream, Roy is helping Albert move house from one location to another. Moving house is a big undertaking, one of the most stressful things we can do. Roy loads the van with Albert, and also drives it, so the burden of this move is shared, and Albert has great support, in theory.

This is a Shadow dream, so Roy Keane represents an aspect of Albert's character that is literally in the shadows, that has been rejected, or hasn't been used in Albert's daily life for whatever reason.

I wonder what qualities Albert sees in Roy Keane. Roy is a very talented man. He is the Irish football assistant manager, and one of the greatest Irish professional footballers. He is courageous, has a no-nonsense approach, is practical, stands on his dignity, doesn't suffer fools gladly, frightens people with his stare, is touchy, has a chip on his shoulder, is emotional and honest, has a warm heart behind a tough exterior, loves his dogs, and is an admirable carrier of masculinity. As a well-known public figure, these are just some of the perceptions we have about him, and presumably Albert doesn't know Roy Keane personally any more than we do. Whatever qualities Albert sees in Roy are the qualities that are 'driving his stuff'.

Albert goes on to say, 'No matter how much we loaded the van, the flat never emptied.' So there's a lot of baggage there to get rid of from where Albert lives. It's as if he's unable to get rid of his past, which seems to be never ending. This dream is asking Albert to pay attention to his baggage, and to start to deal with it in the way that Roy Keane would – to bring the positive, masculine qualities he sees in Roy to bear on his baggage. If he lives those qualities out in his life, what he is dealing with can eventually be brought to an end.

If possible Albert should go and talk to someone he trusts and they will help to relieve him of the unending heavy burden that the dream points to. And it is wonderfully hopeful that Albert has inside him such an iconic figure of masculinity as Roy Keane to help him get the job done. By bringing all of those qualities out of the shadows and into the light, his Shadow will strengthen him on his psychological journey towards maturity, and help him cope with the immediate task at hand in a focused manner.

Nessa's dream of Madonna and Nicole Kidman

✦ ✧ ✦ ✧ ✦

I had a dream where Madonna was playing in the local playground in my village. Then the dream jumped to me getting Nicole Kidman's hair caught in my mouth. It was a weird dream, but not a bad dream. I feel like I can still feel the hair in my mouth. – Nessa

✦ ✧ ✦ ✧ ✦

Nessa's dream presents her with two images of womanhood. They are both celebrities and both actresses: Madonna and Nicole Kidman. Since they are of the same sex as Nessa, this can be characterised as a Shadow dream and, as is more usual than not in a woman's case, this is a collective dream because there are two Shadow figures.

Nessa says, 'Madonna was playing in the local playground in my village'. Play is a very creative activity, particularly for young children, because it is how they learn. 'Then the dream jumped to me getting Nicole Kidman's hair caught in my mouth.' So the movement is from being an observer of Madonna to actually having Nicole Kidman's hair caught in her mouth, which is a very intimate form of touching, or indeed tasting. Usually it's your own long hair that gets caught in your mouth. Very young children and infants in the playground use their mouths to bite in order to explore and get to know their world.

Play can also mean a theatrical or music performance, and here Nessa says 'Madonna was playing in the local playground in my village'. The name 'Madonna' is also a reference to the mother of God, so Nessa is describing a visitation by a Goddess, who has appeared in the humble surroundings of a local playground in her village. This tells us that the dream is an important one, and Nessa has been chosen for this privilege.

In the dream, Madonna gives way to Nicole Kidman. The repetition of a female motif shows that there's an equivalence between both figures, and that the same message is being repeated.

What can we say about Madonna and Nicole Kidman, and what do they have in common? What sort of Shadow qualities do they express that Nessa needs and could be trying to incorporate from her dream? They are successful, beautiful and powerful. As a singer, Madonna is a superstar, and singing is an expression of the deepest feeling: Madonna communicates through her voice. She's also a dancer and knows how to use her body to express emotion. As an actress, Nicole Kidman also knows how to express emotion; she does so through her eyes on screen, even as she presents a cool exterior, which Madonna also has. Through their very public break-ups with Guy Ritchie and Tom Cruise, both women have shown how women deal with adversity, and also get what they want.

Madonna and Nicole Kidman are entertainers who also play at being women. They show how to present the image of being the woman. And Nessa can obviously take lessons from these two master manipulators of the image.

As Nessa says, 'It was a weird dream, but not a bad dream.' As we saw in Aidan's dream of Paloma Faith, the original meaning of the word 'weird' was to have the power to control the fate of men, as seen in Shakespeare's three 'Weird Sisters' in *Macbeth* or the three 'Fates' or goddesses of Greek mythology who controlled human destiny. So it looks as if Nessa has joined this pantheon with Madonna and Nicole Kidman! She can learn from the experts in being a woman who knows what she wants and they can become a formidably weird – but not bad – trio who control the fate of men. She should go out and play in the playground of life as the very confident woman – or goddess – that her unconscious is offering her.

Finally, Nessa says, 'I feel like I can still feel the hair in my mouth.' This is the lingering effect of this dream. Hair traditionally symbolises virility and strength, and as an important woman's attribute, it signifies seduction. What feeling does the sensation of hair in her mouth leave her with? Is it a feeling of distaste? Or a feeling of being touched by greatness, and being exceptionally honoured? Maybe both are true. She needs to recognise the feeling and name it, because that feeling is also a part of this dream. In any case Nessa should live her inner Madonna and continue to become an intimate of Nicole Kidman!

Brian's dream of getting into a fight, but not being able to hit

✦ ✧ ✦ ✧ ✦

I dream that I get into a fight, but I can't hit. I can't move my arms fast and I have no strength. I'm full of fear and anticipate a lot of pain from the other guy. – Brian

✦ ✧ ✦ ✧ ✦

*B*rian begins by saying, 'I dream …', using the present tense, demonstrating that for him this dream is a living reality, which is the appropriate way to approach this expression of his unconscious. 'I dream …' also implies that Brian dreams a version of the dream regularly.

This is a Shadow dream because the other guy in Brian's dream is a Shadow figure of himself, revealing an aspect of himself that he doesn't recognise or acknowledge. And when faced with the Shadow, Brian says, 'I'm full of fear, and anticipate a lot of pain from the other guy.'

The Shadow is made up of aspects of ourselves that were rejected because they were unacceptable to our parental figures, and these qualities contain a lot of unused potential; a lot of energy – if we could only harness their potential. In Brian's case, he's fighting his own Shadow figure, which represents this aspect of himself that has been jettisoned. As he gets into the fight, he's afraid that he's going to be overwhelmed: 'I can't hit', he says, 'I can't move my arms fast, and I have no strength.'

This is typical of the way we feel often about the Shadow: our house is divided against itself. The immobility in the face of such a powerful force is also a typical motif from nightmares, when the part of the brain that prohibits movement while we're asleep takes charge of the psyche, and brings this mechanism to our attention.

The Shadow aspects in our personalities that remain unused are going to cause us pain when we start to exercise them again and bring them back into use. So from the drama of the dream, what are the qualities that this 'other guy' – the Shadow – has? What are we told about him?

This Shadow figure knows how to fight. And he also knows how to win. Unlike Brian, he can hit; he can move his arms fast, and he has strength. He can also inflict a lot of pain. So he's a warrior. The warrior is very powerful, and while a warrior only fights as a last resort, he continues to train and exercise for an eventuality that he hopes will never happen.

An aggressive Shadow figure often compensates for an overly passive personality in our waking life. So Brian should begin to use the fighting qualities that will turn him into a winner in his everyday. These qualities are all there in potential in his unconscious, and if he consciously brings them back into use, they'll stop attacking him in him dreams, and they will also lose their nightmarish qualities. But most importantly, Brian will also be a winner in his life because of using them!

Maeve's dream of two people hanging from a tree

✦ ✧ ✦ ✧ ✦

I keep having a dream of two people hanging from a tree. They are dressed all in black. –
Maeve

✦ ✧ ✦ ✧ ✦

To be dressed all in black is an indicator of the Shadow, so Maeve has had a Shadow dream, which indicates part of the personality which is split off, repressed or denigrated. All aspects of this dream are expressions of herself.

In the United States, following the emancipation of slaves until as late as the 1960s, lynch mobs used to hang African Amercian men and women from trees in order to intimidate that population. A similar thing happened in Ireland: rebels were hung from trees as a warning to others, particularly during the Williamite wars of the late seventeenth century, and again after the 1798 rebellion.

So this is also a warning dream that draws on collective historical memory in order to intimidate Maeve – to frighten her into doing nothing about a manifest injustice. All silence is deadly: it allows abusers to triumph. So Maeve is going to have to overcome her natural reluctance and courageously speak out. She's going to have to deal with what this Shadow dream is presenting to her by first examining the main image in the dream from every possible angle.

Two people are hanging from a tree dressed in black, the colour of mourning. The image is doubled, which, as well as laying emphasis on the collective level of the psyche as opposed to the individual, also suggests ambivalence, and two conflicting points of view.

The two people in a person's life that come from the collective level of the unconscious are our parents. And in Maeve's dream she has them swinging from a tree. This is also a Shadow dream, so it is drawing on Maeve's qualities that haven't seen the light of day, or that are incompatible with the orthodox view of life: qualities that perhaps Maeve has had to repress out of fear of displeasing her parents. These forbidden qualities that she may have acquiesced in splitting off from because she wanted to be a good girl are asking to be brought back to life in her personality – hence, the conflict.

As a conscious adult, Maeve has to examine the strictures that came from her parents and teachers to see if they still hold true. In a sense she has to triumph over her parental figures and their outlook, maybe even as she has done in the drama of her dream by metaphorically killing them, and the authoritative attitudes they represent.

It could also be that this dream is a way for Maeve to express the unthinkable, and satisfy a death wish she has against her parents. Whatever it is, the presentation of this dream is asking Maeve to take it out of the shadows and to face up to it.

Maeve needs to inhabit who she is, the good with the bad, and become a unique individual. She must use all of the qualities she possesses including her Shadow aspects that may be awkward and undeveloped as yet, acknowledging the parts of her personality that she finds unacceptable and that she would prefer weren't a part of her make-up. We all say of some people, 'I'd like to kill them', but we don't actually mean it; we use the phrase figuratively. Maeve should fire on all cylinders using her good impulses as well as the bad, employing the energy tied up in the bad in as productive a way as is possible. Eventually Maeve will soar into the air under her own steam, and won't need to be hung out to dry if she becomes a rebel, nor have to aggressively triumph over those who would oppose or inhibit her just because they can, frightening her into silence and submission.

3
Self Dreams

*T*he God-like archetype called the Self is the organising genius behind the total personality, and it's experienced as being radically other and awe-inspiring. It's like language, which is a perfect manifestation of the Self, and which comes from that other place outside of consciousness. The Self is responsible for implementing the blueprint of life through each stage of our life cycle – each act of the hero's journey – and for bringing about the best adjustment that individual circumstances will allow, in order for us to realise our potential as human beings, to cope with the normal stresses of life, to work productively and fruitfully, and finally, to make a contribution to our community. The goal of the Self is wholeness, or well-being. There's a Hebrew word for it: '*shalom*'. It means the attainment of the fullest possible Self-realisation in the psyche and in the world.

When the Self appears in dreams, it often indicates a need for stabilisation or ordering. The Self manifests in dreams as that circular castle in the centre of the square, which is a mandala image used in Buddhism and other religions as a representation of the universe, held to symbolise a striving for unity and completeness. The Self can be personified in dreams as the president, king or queen, or can be projected onto supra-personal entities such as the state, the sun, nature, the universe, God or the human voice with the divine power to create words and communicate.

The Self is an inner guiding factor different from consciousness. It is the regulating centre of the unconscious that brings about a constant extension and maturing of our personality. In a man's dreams it may be personified as a guru, a wise old man or a spirit of nature. In a woman's dreams it may be personified as a superior female figure – a priestess, earth mother or a goddess of nature or of love.

The power and authority that the Self brings for the dreamer carry the energy needed to undertake great change. Self dreams occur when a person is at a crossroads or turning point in their life. Ultimately the Self leads towards an accumulation of wisdom and, finally, acceptance.

Timothy's dream of being elected president

✦ ✧ ✦ ✧ ✦

I had a dream last night where I was elected president. I didn't know I was running for it, and I couldn't figure out if I was happy with it or not. – Timothy

✦ ✧ ✦ ✧ ✦

What a wonderful dream: Timothy for President! The organising principle of the personality is the Self. It's an archetype, or a universal pattern or motif, which is running like a hard drive in our unconscious. It unites the disparate elements of the personality into a whole, giving the person a sense of 'oneness' and firmness. When a person says he's in the zone and feels in harmony with himself and the world, the Self archetype is performing its work correctly!

Consequently, the Self often personifies in dreams as a king or queen, or as in this dream, as president. Timothy has been raised to the highest office in the land. In psychological terms, when Timothy allows the archetype of the Self to do its work, a sense of wholeness is brought to his personality.

This process of being elected president happened to Timothy unconsciously: 'I didn't know I was running for it'. Timothy's unconscious has taken over, and subjected him to being president in order to unite his personality. What is pictured in the dream is just a proposal from Timothy's unconscious: until Timothy gives his conscious assent, it is not a done deal. All dreams have to take consciousness into account as well, so that a new, third position arrives, which partakes of both the unconscious and consciousness.

Timothy is required to consciously take that unconscious subjection and turn it around so that he can voluntarily take charge of it and own it. Thereby he will become a free subject, a free individual, who willingly embraces the order, organisation and unification proposed by his unconscious. And I think that's why the dream uses the symbol of President, as opposed to the Queen of England, for example, who rules over her subjects. The President of the Republic is the first among equals, which is what Timothy has to become: a free individual, pursuing his own ends and ideas; a subject of the Self, rather than being subjected to the Self.

Since Timothy has had such a dream about the Self, it suggests that whatever is happening in his daily life needs the organisation that the Self can supply. This is why the Self has appeared to him so clearly in his dream. So it's worth Timothy examining his daily life to see whether he is in danger of fragmentation from some activity in which he is engaged, and which goes against the Self.

There's another danger here that arises from identifying with the Self. Timothy could become over-inflated, even deluded, developing what's known as a 'mana personality'. This is where a man identifies with the archetype of the Wise Old Man and believes that he is so exceptional that he has superior insight for mankind, or where a woman becomes the Great Mother, ready to nourish the world. However, Timothy expresses his cautious ambivalence in the dream when he says, 'I couldn't figure out if I was happy with it or not', which certainly sounds humble and grounded, and paves the way for him to accept or to reject what his unconscious is proposing.

The elevation in status described in this dream also means that, at some level, Timothy has to move from being a private citizen to becoming a public statesman, with all of the responsibilities that entails. The dream is a beautiful metaphor for accepting maturity and growing up. So Timothy should embrace it because by accepting the mature responsibilities that are offered to him in the course of his life as he knows it, his overall good and completeness now and in the future will be assured. He will become a wise leader, which is both the internal and external goal of the hero's journey, in that he can bring some treasure back to the community. Timothy is being offered a great vocation, so he should give it real consideration and decide whether he is up for the challenge and the difficulties that accepting such an individual journey entails.

Ultan's dream of being invited to dinner with the emperor of China

✦ ✧ ✦ ✧ ✦

I dreamt that myself and my family were invited to dinner with a guy and his family. I imagine he was the emperor of China as the place was grand and he seemed important. I'm not thinking about travelling to China. – Ultan

✦ ✧ ✦ ✧ ✦

The other side of the world, or the dream location, if you like, can often appear in dreams as China or the orient. This shows that the dream comes from an unconscious place that we experience as being other, or alien. So in his dream, Ultan is 'invited to dinner with a guy and his family', who he imagines was the emperor of China because, as he says, 'the place was grand and he seemed important'.

While Ultan may not be thinking about travelling to China, he did travel to China in his dream. When dealing with the unconscious, he needs to accept what that represents as a fact of psychic experience, and let it permeate his consciousness.

China is an enormous country, and this representative of the Chinese empire and his family – this representative of the whole of the unconscious, if you like – invited Ultan and his family to dine with him; to break bread with him, to share. And Ultan is correct, this is a very important invitation indeed. He is being asked to allow the magnitude of his powerful unconscious to participate in his conscious life, and to contribute the insights and the direction that such a prestigious invitation can open up for him and his family.

Ultan's dream is a wonderfully stabilising one, because the emperor of China represents Ultan's real Self, the organising principle of his whole personality, what the Greeks used to call his 'daimon', and the Romans his 'genius'. And the fact that the Self has appeared in his dream and issued him with such an important invitation means that he is being required to ground himself, and allow that other, which he experiences as the emperor of China, to have a say in his life, and to follow the direction that arises from the contemplation of such a divine figure. The fact that the last emperor of China, Henry Puyi, died in 1967 emphasises the symbolic nature of this function in Ultan's dream, and also in his daily life, because this dream needs to be honoured consciously.

Ultan's dreams over the coming months will be very important, as the effects of this invitation are turned into an ongoing reality. He must pay attention to them and take them on board. To paraphrase Sigmund Freud, Ultan's dream of having dinner with the emperor of China is literally the royal road to the unconscious. And if it's possible for him, Ultan might consider undergoing a psychoanalysis, which would allow as much of the unconscious into his conscious life as he could bear. In the light of his extraordinary dream, such a massive contribution could only work for his good.

4

Animal Dreams

*T*he Self as the guiding centre of our personalities is often symbolised as an animal in dreams, which represents our instinctive nature and our connectedness with the land and our surroundings. That is why there are so many helpful animals in myths and fairy tales. The animal motif is usually symbolic of man's primitive and instinctive nature. However, the animal that lives in man's instincts may become dangerous if it is not recognised and integrated into his life so that its primitive nature can be tamed.

We can control instincts by our will, but we are also able to suppress, distort and wound them. When an animal is hurt and wounded it can be dangerous and wild, and certainly not subject to reason. It's also possible for suppressed instincts to gain control of us, to suddenly take over us, and even to bring about our destruction – so they have a Shadow aspect as well. These suppressed instincts threaten civilised man when the animal within is alienated from its true nature.

The animals that appear in our dreams deserve to be given the greatest attention, so that instead of threatening us, they can

share with us their many gifts, and remind us how to properly
harness our instinctual energy.

Bridget's dream of a cake full of rats

✦ ✧ ✦ ✧ ✦

I had a dream the other night where I was slicing a cake and when I cut through it, it was full of dead rats! What the flip, lads?! – Bridget

✦ ✧ ✦ ✧ ✦

This is a warning dream for Bridget. A cake is something we enjoy eating, and normally we have it as a treat: we eat a slice of cake to celebrate a birthday or a wedding, to enjoy at Christmas time or to share with friends. When somebody bakes you a cake, it's a very personal gift that nourishes you both physically and emotionally. Bridget says, however, that when she cut through this particular cake, 'it was full of dead rats'.

Rats are not a food that we would eat in the normal run of things, unless we were starving. Rats are vermin, they bring disease, and they are the very opposite of something loving, enjoyable and fun. The rats in Bridget's dream were dead and decomposing. Bridget gives her reaction in a question: 'What the flip, lads?' In other words, what's happening; what's going on here? Is this dream lacking in seriousness and playing games with her? Is it being somehow being disrespectful or even impertinent?

I think the dream is having a bit of fun at Bridget's expense. It paints a picture that cake isn't something she should be eating, for whatever reason – maybe she is on a diet, or has to watch her sugar intake; we don't know. But the bottom line in this dream is that what she expects to be pleasurable and enjoyable doesn't turn out that way, and she's taken unawares by the nasty surprise.

There are distant echoes here of the traditional children's nursery rhyme 'Sing a Song of Sixpence' in the lines, 'When the pie was opened/The birds began to sing'. And more recently from the Robert Aldrich film *What Ever Happened to Baby Jane?*, which has a horrific scene in which Bette Davis serves Joan Crawford her lunch, and Crawford lifts the lid to find a dead rat inside. Bridget's dream borrows these motifs and serves up the hard lesson that her expectations can be cruelly dashed. The dream attempts to shock her into seeing how easily one reality can change into another, which is a typical Trickster motif – that is Bridget's warning in this dream. So she should examine where in her life she is being over-optimistic, too trusting perhaps, and be prepared for the eventuality that life can let her down when she least expects it, shapeshifting into its opposite and dashing her expectations.

There's an even stronger warning in the dramatic horror of this dream. It just isn't possible for Bridget to take in or to digest the reality presented to her in the cake. It's something so horrific and abhorrent that she deliberately minimises it by her 'What the flip, lads?' remark. Sometimes the reality that we crash into has something of the uncanny about it that we cannot assimilate, or that we're just not able to cope with. Maybe the dream is pointing her towards something that has happened already in her life since the rats are already dead. Has somebody betrayed her, ratted on her, informed on her, let her down, behaved disloyally towards her, or deserted a cause that she believed in, which resulted in such a hurt that it gnaws at her like a rat? If this is indeed the case for Bridget, I would suggest she could be helped by talking through it with a professional. Since the dream has served up this meal for her attention, her unconscious seems to think that now is the time to deal with it, and that she is now in possession of the proper resources to deal with the aftermath.

Dermot's dream of pigeons pooping on him

❖ ✦ ❖ ✦

Sometimes I dream that pigeons keep pooping on me. I'm running around trying to dodge it.
– Dermot

✦ ❖ ✦ ❖ ✦

*D*ermot says he has this dream 'sometimes', meaning now and then, occasionally or at times. So he's saying that this is a reccurring dream. The reason for this repetition is that the message the dream is trying to illustrate hasn't been taken on board by him, yet the message is very simple.

The drama of the dream clearly shows that Dermot is literally being shat upon, and that he is 'running around trying to dodge it', as he says. In the dream this action is done by pigeons, but I think there's a pun here: a pigeon is slang for a dupe, which is an easily gullible person. In the late seventeenth century, 'to pigeon' meant to trick or swindle a person at cards. And in the betting world, rogues and their dupes are referred to as 'rooks and pigeons'. Interestingly, a 'poop' is another word for an ineffectual or stupid person, a fool, perhaps an abbreviation of 'nincompoop'. So there's a verbal doubling-up or condensation here, where all the meanings in several chains of association ultimately converge on a single idea in the dream, to underline the point that Dermot is being taken for an 'eejit', to the extent that people 'keep pooping' on him, as he says.

In everyday language, a party pooper is a person whose behaviour or attitude spoils other people's enjoyment. And the dream seems to have been triggered by people who attribute so little value to Dermot that they're behaving badly towards him, treating him as an idiot, and robbing him of the quiet enjoyment he has a right to. That says much more about them than it does about Dermot. Nevertheless, the dream has brought this situation to Dermot's consciousness time and time again, and he hasn't been listening. So by painting this picture of pooping pigeons, the dream emphatically demands that Dermot pay attention to what's happening.

Dermot should examine what's going on around him, because the dream is a representation of what has registered in his unconscious, even if he wasn't consciously aware of this situation before, or maybe he did pick up something out of the corner of his eye. In any case, a dream brings to his attention something that he hasn't fully acknowledged up to now, and in this dream it has poked a little fun at him to win his attention.

When he has identified the people who are treating him badly, he should stand up for his rights, and hand the poop right back because it doesn't belong to him: the poop belongs to them, and he wouldn't want to be considered a thief now, would he? He certainly shouldn't waste his valuable time 'running around trying to dodge it'. A picture has been painted for him by his unconscious, clearly pointing out that his behaviour is ineffectual and stupid in this regard, and his way of dealing with the problem isn't working. If he is being treated badly, he needs to say so unambiguously, and to confront the bad behaviour of others head on so that it can be brought to an end. There's a principle at work here: never reward bad behaviour.

If he feels that he can't confront his abusers, then he should chalk it up to experience and move on, leaving the bullies behind. Certainly it's a waste of time trying to house-train other people and getting them to change their attitudes towards him, unless they have the capacity for insight, and the potential willingness to change their unacceptable behaviour.

The bottom line from Dermot's dream is that being pooped upon and running around trying to avoid the poop must be brought to an end, because as a human being it's unworthy of him. At a minimum, Dermot deserves to be treated properly.

Kate's dream of a white snake

✦ ✧ ✦ ✧ ✦

A few weeks ago I had a dream about a giant white snake. The snake was in my home. I was afraid of it at first, but I eventually entered the room it was in to try and kill it using a steel ruler. I then woke up so I have no idea if I won or the snake did. – Kate

✦ ✧ ✦ ✧ ✦

We have an inherent fear of snakes, which seems to be bred into our collective unconscious. Snakes signify danger. And in this dream, a giant white snake was in Kate's home, which is an inappropriate place for it. But the movement in the dream is to face the threat head on instead of running away. Kate says, 'I entered the room it was in to try and kill it using a steel ruler.' So important work is being done in this dream: the dreamer is facing her fears, and she's dealing with the dangerous problem.

In mythological terms, a snake is a symbol of transcendence – literally climbing over or beyond, of surmounting – or going beyond limits. It also symbolises the potential for poison or for healing, since it represents the therapeutic symbol of the Roman god of medicine Asclepius. A staff with a snake curled around it, which has survived to modern times as a sign of the medical profession, signifies the potential to kill or to cure. In snake-handling cults of initiation, it demonstrates a means of proving yourself. So there's ambiguity here in the use of this symbol in Kate's dream.

A snake grows by shedding its skin. When a snake becomes too big for its skin, it leaves the old skin behind. This marks a transition, indicating a period of change when a person outgrows certain attitudes or ways of dealing with things that may have worked for them in the past but that now should be let go if the person is to grow and mature.

This is an important dream showing a well-known symbol from mythology, and Kate is being encouraged to wake up to the situation that's presented in it, which is a battle to the death. She says, 'I then woke up, so I have no idea if I won or the snake did.' The outcome of the struggle with the snake, a struggle about maturity, can go either way.

Kate must bring her waking consciousness to bear on what her unconscious has presented. She needs to kill her old, outworn attitudes. In the dream she does so, interestingly, with a steel ruler. There's a pun in the language used here. When we are in charge of our own life, we are the 'ruler' of our domain. So she is putting order on the situation with a steely backbone – the snake within, if you like, is the brain stem, the upward growth of the spinal cord. And, fortunately, Kate isn't afraid to carry out this task. All in all, the battle with the snake – again, perhaps there's a pun about something venomous, deceitful or treacherous – has the potential for a very successful outcome.

Finally, Freud said that all dreams have a sexual component, so a 'giant white snake' could also represent a giant white penis. From this perspective, the symbol of the male sexual organ was in Kate's home, where she lives, and she acknowledges that she was afraid of it at first. But eventually she entered the room where this sexual symbol was present 'to try to kill it using a steel ruler'.

Kate's intention was to kill the snake, but the language she used can also be applied to her fear – to try to kill her fear using a steel ruler. That seems to imply a steely attitude to keep her ambivalent fears around sex in check. A more conscious and balanced attitude would recognise the power that sex has in our lives. This is the less uptight approach, which will cut the giant snake down to size.

The fearsome power of the snake can be destructive in certain circumstances, particularly if Kate dams it up with a steely response. A more measured and balanced response towards the reality of sex in her own life will work towards her fulfilment. From this sexual perspective, size does matter to the extent that she measures with her inner ruler to direct, guide and regulate appropriately.

The dream is asking Kate to outgrow her previous attitudes to sex and adopt a mature approach based on the reality of sex as she experiences it now. So if she updates her attitudes, they will serve her well going forward.

Doireann's dream of the mouse and the cat

✦ ✧ ✦ ✧ ✦

I had a dream twice that a mouse was running across my pillow while I was asleep. Another time it was a cat. Each time I woke up thinking the animal was actually there. – Doireann

✦ ✧ ✦ ✧ ✦

This is a dream series, in that the first dream is repeated in order to ask Doireann to pay attention to it. Then there's a development in the third dream where the animal changes.

Animals represent the instinctual part of our nature, so it is important for us to explore the associations we have to them. In her dream Doireann talks about two of them. She says, 'I had a dream that a mouse was running across my pillow while I was asleep. Another time it was a cat.'

Animals that appear in our dreams are generally there to help us. In mythology they often help the hero to accomplish his or her task. In medieval times a person's soul was supposed to pass at death as a mouse. In medieval superstition the cat was known as a 'familiar', a servant spirit of witches. In symbolism the mouse is indicative of timidity, while the cat represents stealthy cunning, agility and even clairvoyance. So while these creatures are representative of the animal part of our natures, they also have a spiritual aspect. Doireann needs to pay attention to the many levels and qualities that these particular animals are showing to her. She can decide whether they could be a help or a hindrance if she were to incorporate their qualities consciously into her personality.

What do we say about a mouse? We use the phrases 'as quiet as a mouse', 'as timid as a mouse', or 'as tiny as a mouse'. We refer to someone who hides away in the countryside as a 'country mouse'. We also say that tea or soup is strong enough to 'trot a mouse on', meaning that the tread of a mouse is delicate.

And what do we say about a cat? We describe something as 'cat' when it's awful. We talk about a catty or spiteful remark, and use the phrases 'letting the cat out of the bag', a 'fat cat', 'behaving like a scalded cat', 'looking like something the cat brought in', or 'no room to swing a cat', and so on. A cat is bigger than a mouse and almost the opposite to it too in that we don't seem to say good things about cats. There's a lot of information in the language that we use, and all of these associations to the cat and mouse are relevant to Doireann's dream. Only she can assent to the ones that have a personal relevance for her.

Let's put the two animals together, which is what Doireann did in her dream: the same scenario of two different animals 'running across my pillow while I was asleep'. What do we mean when we say that someone is playing 'cat and mouse'? We mean they're playing hard to get, that there is a game going on reminiscent of the way that a cat plays with a mouse, toying with a weaker party, trifling with somebody's affections; or from the mouse's perspective, they're being wary of somebody.

Bearing in mind that this is a dream series that incorporates a development, the most obvious interpretation dramatised by this series is the saying 'While the cat's away, the mouse will play'. In the first two dreams Doireann is shown a mouse at play. In the third dream the cat appears, so that there can be no more playing, and the mouse is absent. Traditionally the mouse and the cat are seen as mortal enemies, so the dream series is pointing to a split in Doireann's personality, whereby she compartmentalises her ability to play, which the dream says can be completely curtailed in certain circumstances.

What does the inhibiting factor of the cat represent for her? Is it the strictures of her partner, her parents or some ideology? It is important to bring more balance into her personality, where whatever is holding her in check can be experienced in a more relaxed fashion – and the mouse and the cat, which represent different aspects of her personality, can both have their say.

It's also important to point out that the mouse and the cat are out of place here. They shouldn't be running across Doireann's pillow while she's asleep. So she needs to wake up to this situation and pay attention to something that's happening behind her back. The dream is repeated twice so it must be a situation in which she needs to take action urgently, and bring whatever it is that's inappropriate to an end.

Emer's dream of the giant spiders

✦ ✧ ✦ ✧ ✦

I dreamt that I was in a huge bathroom. Suddenly these giant spiders appeared and started to attack me. Their eyes were red and they were really hairy. – Emer

✦ ✧ ✦ ✧ ✦

Arachnophobia is an abnormal fear of spiders, and it's more common than we would imagine. If Emer suffers from this, then her dream is terrifying indeed.

A bathroom is a private space where we deal with bodily functions, so Emer is telling us through her dream that she's being attacked in an area that is very personal to her. She says the attackers are giant spiders, presumably with four pairs of legs (or arms), and as Emer describes, with red eyes and are really hairy.

Emer says she's being attacked by 'giant spiders' – plural – so the attack comes from the collective level of the unconscious, which is often the way that a woman's Shadow appears in dreams. So from that Shadow perspective, Emer is being attacked by a part of herself that she has split from, that's undeveloped, and that she considers to be at the primitive level of insects.

We sometimes use the word 'insect' as an epithet meaning a contemptible, insignificant or loathsome person, so it's clear how Emer regards this aspect of herself.

Since this attack is coming from the collective level of the unconscious – at one remove from the personal and individual level – it could even be an attack from her mother, who is one generation back. This possibility could be at work, attacking Emer and undermining her, because the all-enveloping, smothering mother can appear in dreams as a spider.

All dreams also have a sexual component, and from that perspective, I think it's not a massive jump to see Emer wrestling with a sexual assault: an engorged red penis and pubic hair. And if you incorporate the old wives' tale that spiders are venomous and they inject venom into their victims, then being bitten by sex is something that could be terrifying Emer.

The fact that she describes many insects attacking her shows, at a very primitive, instinctual level, that Emer is experiencing this attack as an infestation. She is so split off from this aspect of her personality that it's working against her, and in the dream it's actually attacking her.

Emer needs to figure out where she's being attacked, and what she's reacting to so violently inside. A good clue for all dreams is to examine the previous 24 hours to find out if something could have triggered the dream in the first place.

The normal question about the Shadow – and these spiders are a manifestation of that rejected energy – is: what qualities can the Shadow contribute to the dreamer's personality? Symbolically, spiders have represented patience, and creative powers. They also symbolise cruelty, because the females are dangerous to the males during mating rituals. Again, the dream could be holding up a mirror image. The spiders' aggression, which is experienced as attacking the dreamer, in reality could be an expression of her own impulses, from which she has split off and doesn't acknowledge. Could it be that like spiders, she too is a predator, dangerous to males in sexual situations?

Perhaps the spiders appear in a form so alien and frightening for Emer that she can't verbalise their positive qualities, much less to incorporate their contribution. So Emer will have to wait until she has another dream of animals that are a little further up the food chain in order to relate to them.

On a hopeful note, while not minimising the undoubted importance of Emer's reaction to her dream, in reality spiders in the bathroom are something that people are able to deal with, and normally the spiders are disposed of quite easily. That reality will happen for Emer too, as she consciously plays around with and becomes familiar with the images in this dream, and honours the dream's presence in her life as a psychic fact.

5

Sex and Relationship Dreams

*T*he extravert and the introvert have different attitudes towards relating. The energy flow of the extravert is outwards towards other people. Extraverts take enormous delight in relating to other people, and in relating to new ideas and strange situations. The introvert's energy flow is in the opposite direction, and the primary relationship is with his own subjectivity and inner world. The reality of having to relate to other people provokes a negative response in the introvert until his security is assured, and only then can he give his assent to engage with people, however reluctantly.

Relationship dreams reveal the area of growth that's needed in our personalities. Both the extravert and the introvert are presented with a drama that cultivates the opposite attitude to their comfort zone. This brings about a greater balance in their personalities. Relationship dreams demand that we be able to move back and forwards between both of those poles – extraverted and introverted – in a way that works towards achieving wholeness.

As a very general rule, women tend to concern themselves with the nature of relationships and with relating, while men tend to appear to be more concerned with the nature of being, which Shakespeare portrayed brilliantly in Hamlet's 'To be, or not to be …' speech. Even young girls tend to be more affiliative and to seek social interaction, while boys are more task oriented.

This, too, is often illustrated in sex and relationship dreams, often pointing towards surprising conclusions that challenge the orthodoxies we subscribe to. For example, dreams show that sex is always experienced at some level as traumatic. Dreams can assert that anatomy doesn't necessarily determine our identities: masculinity and femininity are more symbolic positions that we assume. Sex dreams show that these symbolic positions are never completely settled, so that they're a source of ongoing questioning in our dreams. Dreams also point out that our sexual desire isn't determined by the opposite sex, but by something else. There are many implications about sex with which our unconscious will upset us.

While such images in our dreams can cause us great distress and confusion initially, it's important to remember that by engaging consciously with the perplexing images proposed by our unconscious in our relationship and sex dreams, and especially by putting them into words despite embarrassment or even disgust, we'll be more able to express the full truth of ourselves going forward. We'll also orient ourselves around sex and relationships in keeping with our eternal unconscious desire, rather than being ruled by societal norms which change over time.

Deirdre's sex dreams about her male friend

✦ ✧ ✦ ✧ ✦

I keep having sex dreams about my male friend. He is gay and I'm really getting attached to him in the dream. I've told him and we laugh about it, but what's the story? – Deirdre

✦ ✧ ✦ ✧ ✦

Sex is the most intimate connection we can make with another human being. So the sex dreams Deirdre has about her male friend are about being intimately connected with him; as Deirdre herself says: 'I'm really getting attached to him in the dream'. The developmental history of the word 'keep' that Deirdre employs – 'I keep having sex dreams' – shows that it once meant to gape or give heed in watching, which was a figurative extension of laying hold of. The word also meant to stand out and be visible. So the sexual sub-text in all these associations is clear.

Deirdre's confusion as described in her dream seems to be caused by the fact that her male friend is gay. 'What's the story?' she asks. In other words, why is she having sex dreams about a male friend who is gay and presumably isn't available to her in a sexual way? Deirdre's words in her opening sentence are, 'I keep having sex dreams about my male friend.' The important factor here is that her friend is a man. So Deirdre fancies him, and there's nothing wrong in that; her impulse is normal. It's only in the second sentence that we learn 'he is gay'.

It is such a pity that her gay male friend can't respond in the way that Deirdre desires. While Deirdre can be emotionally intimate with him, and share her dreams with him, it's important that she has straight, male friends in her life as well, so that she can take the sexual intimacy with a man that is dramatised in her dream to someone who can give her what she desires.

We can see that the dream brings her attention to the fact that she needs that particular outlet as well, since Deirdre has told her gay friend that she's having sex dreams about him, which is a probing appeal to his heterosexual side, a come-on she immediately downplays: 'I've told him, and we laugh about it'. Presumably he hasn't taken the heterosexual bait, otherwise Deirdre would have have mentioned it. And might I point out very gently that what Deirdre is doing in teasing her gay friend with her sexual desires as expressed in her dreams isn't the kindest thing to do. She shouldn't manipulate their friendship, otherwise they will both end up disappointed. That's the real story for Deirdre.

Eileen's dream about her old friend who died

✦ ✧ ✦ ✧ ✦

I dreamt about an old friend last night who died a few years ago. In the dream we were having a very passionate and sexual affair. We were just friends when he was alive. It has really disturbed me. – Eileen

✦ ✧ ✦ ✧ ✦

*I*sn't that a lovely dream to have, where Eileen is visited again by an old friend who has died? Since having sex with someone is the most intimate thing we can do with them, when Eileen says of her friend in the dream, 'we were having a very passionate and sexual affair', she's also talking about having an ongoing, intimate relationship with him. She says, 'We were just friends when he was alive,' so maybe this is a dammed up residue of wanting to be sexually involved with him, which didn't happen at the time for various reasons, and which is finding its expression now in her dreams at a safer time.

Or maybe Eileen is having the dream to connect her with the qualities of her old friend, or the ideals that her friend had held out for her. Death in dreams – manifested here in Eileen's old friend who died – points towards a profound transformation. This dream is mobilising the energy of the qualities she sees in her friend, and asks Eileen to inhabit them, to employ them in her own life, and to strengthen the qualities that she has in embryonic form that her unconscious intuits she needs at this point in her life, including perhaps having a full-blown sexual relationship. Is the dream pointing out to Eileen in an unthreatening way that a sexual relationship, indeed a passionate affair, can be had with someone who can also be her friend?

So while Eileen says that the dream has really disturbed her, I'd say that it is doing no harm. The habitual paths we tread in our lives need to be shaken up from time to time, so that we can create something new. Perhaps travelling in an unexpected direction that will fill out our personalities may be what is required. In Eileen's case, it means using the qualities that she has admired in her friend to give her a new lease of life, to increase her passion, and to disturb the universe somewhat!

Fidelma's dream of going to her ex's house

✦ ◇ ✦ ◇ ✦

I dreamt that I went to my ex's house, who is now married. I wanted to see his mother, who also lives in the house. I wanted to talk to his mother about cooking and wine. Then my ex came in and we went for a walk. He said that things weren't going well with his partner, and she only brings him cakes in bed. We hugged then. We had a difficult break up four years ago, and this has wrecked my head. – Fidelma

✦ ◇ ✦ ◇ ✦

*T*his dream shows Fidelma that some part of her psyche wishes to get back with her ex. She says that they had a difficult break-up four years ago, but that doesn't change the fact that they chose each other to have a relationship with in the first place. So several years ago there was some compatibility there, and that still exists. It's appropriate to mourn the loss of the good parts of a relationship that ended four years ago, even if they were obscured by 'a difficult break-up'. Fidelma probably means that the dream has 'wrecked her head', but you can also read it that the difficult break-up wrecked her head as well, hence her faulty logic in the dream, which is tempting her back towards a further disaster, which would be a regression in more ways than one.

Fidelma's reasoning in the dream for the current relationship of her ex with his new wife is that, as she says, 'his partner only brings him cakes in bed'. The phrase 'cakes and ale' means a good time or filled with pleasure. Furthermore, in this context, the word 'cake' comes from an Indo-European root that means something round and lumpy: in sexual terms, this means breasts and buttocks! So Fidelma posits in her dream that being good in bed is the only reason he married his wife.

This dream is staged to draw Fidelma's attention to something that she hasn't admitted to consciously, so in her dream she goes for a walk with her ex. He tells her things aren't going well with his wife, and they 'hug', which is a word from a Scandinavian source meaning 'to comfort'. A part of Fidelma wants to re-kindle their relationship to be comforted. And she fools herself in the dream by saying, 'I wanted to talk to his mother about cooking and wine,' which is really about contacting the nourishing, mothering part of herself that could cook food for her ex and give him wine to drink. It's certainly more expressive of her warm heart and her personality than limiting a relationship to sex alone! But at this stage in Fidelma's life, it would mean putting new wine in old bottles; adding or imposing something new to an established order. Her ex is also now married with a wife, even though in the dream I note that Fidelma refers to her as 'partner' rather than 'wife'. The results of making such a contact with Fidelma's ex could be disastrous. Already, Fidelma is saying 'this has wrecked my head', so at some level she's acknowledging that truth, which she knows deep down in her soul.

Fidelma is having the dream to warn her about retrospective falsification, of seeing the old relationship through rose-tinted spectacles. It's important for her to remember the bad times in the old relationship as well as pining after the good, and bring some conscious perspective to bear on what the unconscious has presented. In other words, she needs to get a grip! And if she is feeling lonely, she needs to make an effort to find a new relationship, or find some newness in a current relationship, and consign the relationship with her ex to memory and move on, even though those four years would have had an influence on her personality – nothing is ever wasted.

Finally, she must analyse the phrase, 'I wanted to talk to his mother about cooking and wine.' Is that something she used to do, or is it bizarre in the context of his mother? The phrase is certainly expressing a desire to talk to a mother, and also a desire to talk about cooking and wine. So Fidelma should listen to the positive expressions of her personality, and find healthy outlets for them that won't put her or others through further pain and suffering through re-living 'a difficult break-up'. On the evidence of this dream, it might also be useful for Fidelma to talk through that break-up with a therapist or counsellor, and finally put it to bed.

Adam's dream of a girl he really likes

✦ ✧ ✦ ✧ ✦

I had a dream that I was around my home area where there were a few people that I know, including a girl that I really like. I was being sort of rebuffed by them. Then they realised their mistake and approached me to apologise. A thunderstorm came and they ran off except for the girl I like. A volcano erupted and lava started pouring from the sky. She was petrified and held on to me for dear life. We eventually got to safety. – Adam

✦ ✧ ✦ ✧ ✦

Doesn't this dream tell the story of the romantic hero: Adam is rebuffed by the girl he really likes, she realises her mistake and stays with him and finally, he saves the damsel in distress!

The dream begins in Adam's home territory, where he's being snubbed by a few people he knows. He says, 'they realised their mistake, and approached me to apologise.' So the collective in his home area realise the injury that they've done to him and acknowledge it by apologising.

In the middle of the dream there was a catastrophe: 'a thunderstorm came' and 'a volcano erupted and lava started pouring from the sky.' Adam is describing his sexual climax and the creative force of passion, which is in keeping with the underlying theme of this dream. Lava is molten rock, but the word actually comes from the Latin word '*lavare*' to wash, said to be from a river caused by a sudden downpour of rain after a thunderstorm. Adam and the girl he likes are washed by this, baptised if you like, and the girl is 'petrified', meaning she's turned to stone, hardened or solidified. You can hear the undercurrent of sexual imagery continuing. Adam says, 'She ... held onto me for dear life', presumably in sexual congress. Adam concludes, 'We eventually got to safety.' The word 'safety' originally meant redeemed, bought back, paid off, or freed, and only later signified security. So in Adam's dream their love story has moved onto the level of mythology, where our hero and his damsel are redeemed, as symbolised by sex.

Since the drama of this dream delineates a hero's journey, his dream is preparing Adam to be the hero. The energy flowing from these images is being mobilised in his unconscious so that he can pursue this girl he really likes and win her affection. According to his dream, all Adam has to do is acknowledge the heroic, protective qualities that he possesses innately, although perhaps he hasn't used them up to now; and be bold, in all senses of that word, so that he can truly live the dream!

Padraig's constant erotic dreams

◆ ◇ ◆ ◇ ◆

I have constant erotic dreams, with all kinds of people in them, men and women, people I know and strangers. There are orgies, but the people's faces have no expression on them, just blank. Even though they are about sex, I don't wake up aroused. I'm in a relationship.
– Padraig

◆ ◇ ◆ ◇ ◆

*O*ften our unconscious tries to compensate for what's not happening in our conscious life, and Padraig says, 'I have constant erotic dreams … about sex'. Why would that be so?

I wonder if these dreams really 'about sex', as Padraig says, or if there is something else that the dreams are pointing out to him? 'Erotic' is an adjective referring to sexual desire, and I think his dream is staging a drama about that, to bring something important about it to his attention. Could it be that the most important phrase in recounting his dream is 'I don't wake up aroused'?

Sex is the most intimate connection we can make with another human being, and Padraig is having constant dreams about connecting to 'all kinds of people'. Even though he is in a relationship, his dream suggests that at some deep level he is not making an intimate, personal connection that is grounding him.

What's glaringly absent from the way he recounts his dream is any sense that he involves himself in these sexual encounters. I suppose we could read with some contextual validity his opening sentence, 'I have constant erotic dreams, with all kinds of people in them', by removing the comma and deleting the final two words, so that it reads, 'I have constant erotic dreams with all kinds of people'. Maybe that's closer to what Padraig is really saying, in that it's an expression of his desire. But as the sentences stand, it's as if he is an uninvolved observer of pornography, at one remove from the action: 'men and women, people I know and strangers. There are orgies'. Are there, indeed?

Although 'all kinds of people' feature in his erotic dreams, they have the same thing in common: 'their faces have no expression on them, just blank'. As human beings, we use our faces to communicate. We react to desire in the faces of others; that's what really turns us on. There's an absence of desire in Padraig's erotic dreams as he relates them. So Padraig is not being turned on. We use the expression 'shooting blanks' to indicate impotence and, interestingly, he too employs that word 'blank', this time to describe a lack of expression, in another sense, a lack of putting into words, shooting verbal blanks.

These people in his dream don't matter to him really: they're interchangeable bodies going through the motions, like models on a catwalk or actors in pornographic videos. And then after the phrase 'I don't wake up aroused', he adds, 'I'm in a relationship.' Is there a link between those two sentences? Because he is in a relationship, he doesn't wake up aroused, is that it? Or is it that because he doen't wake up aroused, he is in a relationship? Maybe these two sentences are simply neutral statements of fact without implying any connection between them, rather like the neutral way he relates the rest of this dream?

There's certainly more than meets the eye in the dream for Padraig. So he needs to ponder it, play around with it, consider it from many angles, and role play the protagonists in his mind. He is everybody in these constant erotic dreams. The word 'constant' means steadfast, immovable, stable and unvarying, which is the way that we describe our fantasies, particularly the ones that get us to orgasm, or not to orgasm, as the case may be.

If Padraig judges that it's right for him, he should commit to the relationship he is in, and let whatever arises out of the personal associations he brings to his erotic dreams have their say in his sexual life with his partner. He should speak about it, put words on it, give it expression. And if it's not to be, then he should end the relationship in a mature manner that gives his partner respect, and move on eventually to someone who's more compatible, and who engages more of his personality, so that he can be truly stirred up by passion, and not jaded by it.

Rory's erotic dreams never about his girlfriend

✦ ✧ ✦ ✧ ✦

I always have erotic dreams, but never about my girlfriend! I dream about girls I know and even sometimes men are also included in the sex. I love my girlfriend, and don't understand this. – Rory

✦ ✧ ✦ ✧ ✦

Freud said every dream can be viewed from a sexual perspective. And here Rory openly says that he always has erotic dreams, which might suggest that his unconscious tries to compensate for what's not happening in everyday life. As he points out, these erotic dreams are never about his girlfriend. So I wonder what the difficulty is for Rory there: what could his dream be trying to bring to his attention? He says, 'I love my girlfriend, and don't understand this.' Is it because he loves her that he is holding back from placing her in an erotic context? Or is it that his erotic dreams are satisfying aspects that are not being catered for by his girlfriend?

Rory says that he dreams about girls he knows, so he can ask himself what qualities these girls have that his girlfriend lacks. He further says that sometimes men are also included in the sex. So he recognises that he has a bisexual component in his personality.

However, what we seek in sex isn't gendered. So it's possible to say that we have both heterosexual and homosexual components in our personalities. Normally one predominates over the other in our late teens or our early twenties, and we lead with that, while the other normally sinks into the background, where it remains unless our personality needs it.

Which one predominates in Rory's personality? Or maybe I've misunderstood, and he is saying that the men in his erotic dreams are engaged in heterosexual sex. Could it be that he has been feeding his erotic imagination with too much porn? If so, maybe he should cool it for a while. Rory knows the answers to these questions, but needs to ask them of himself.

He says, 'I love my girlfriend, and don't understand this.' Maybe the first step towards understanding is to accept his erotic dreams, in addition to his love for his girlfriend. His unconscious is bringing something to his attention for a reason, something that he hasn't paid attention to before. His unconscious is bringing him new information in the dream, and only he can determine what the particular reason is; the why or the what of that information.

So Rory should be prepared to be surprised by the contribution that his unconscious has brought to him! And as

Carl Jung would say, he should honour the dream and treat it always as a fact of experience, a reality with which he is meant to grapple. He shouldn't be afraid of it, because it will enrich his life in ways he could only dream of.

Seamus's dream of being with a sexy girl in a bar

◆ ✧ ◆ ✧ ◆

I was with a sexy girl in a bar. She took her jeans off. I told her to put them back on, but she wouldn't. I was ordered a drink, and the bar counter was about seven foot tall. – Seamus

◆ ✧ ◆ ✧ ◆

*S*eamus has found himself in a very dangerous situation here. At least Seamus is in a bar, presumably with many other people around, so he can't be accused of sexual assault. In the dream he's acting appropriately by telling the sexy girl to put her jeans back on, but still, it's a situation fraught with danger for him because she refuses to listen to him.

Seamus is having an erotic dream about a sexy girl, but there are warning elements in the dream that are causing him anxiety. It's not a straightforward seduction scene by any means. He says, 'I was ordered a drink', which gives yet another indication that the situation is out of his control: he didn't have a say in what he was drinking. Then he says that 'the bar counter was about seven foot tall'. As well as being a counter in a public house, a bar is also a straight piece of wood or iron, a pole or shaft. In Seamus's dream, it's exaggeratedly long at seven foot, and as a representation of Seamus's desire for the sexy girl, this particular bar probably derives from the physical reaction of his sleeping body while having an erotic dream.

The word 'bar' has other meanings to do with being a barrier, such as to shut out, hinder, prevent, prohibit, obstruct or exclude. These action verbs, when taken in conjunction with the word 'counter' (which has the additional meaning of 'go counter to' or 'oppose'), are warning elements in the dream which should give Seamus pause. The height of the bar counter demonstrates that he's in over his head. The dream points out that the sexy girl is an independent human being with a mind of her own, and Seamus isn't able to control her reckless and dangerous behaviour. These seem to be the messages that are being brought to Seamus's attention.

Seamus needs to bear these lessons in mind in his future encounters with women. He also needs to improve his courtship strategies, re-examine his ability to relate to independent women, realise they are more than just 'sexy', and he shouldn't underestimate them. Seamus must bring his conscious mind to bear on the drama that his unconscious is proposing, and work out a potential strategy for himself going forward. It will be very interesting and instructive to see where he will apply what he has learned from his dream!

Grainne's dream of living with her two brothers and their girlfriends

✦ ✧ ✦ ✧ ✦

I had a dream that I was living with my two brothers and their girlfriends. We were living in a tiny flat, and there were also animals there – pet hamsters and rabbits running around. It was very chaotic and uncomfortable. – Grainne

✦ ✧ ✦ ✧ ✦

A tiny flat, two brothers, two girlfriends, pet hamsters and rabbits running around, and Grainne is living there as well. The environment is not appropriate, and as Grainne says, it's 'very chaotic and uncomfortable'. The dream paints a picture of Grainne and her two brothers living on top of each other, suggesting that she needs space not only for herself, but that she needs to give her brothers space as well.

What do pet hamsters and rabbits do? They have sex – constantly. Grainne is stuck in there with her two brothers and their girlfriends who are having sex in this tiny space, and she has no business being there: she's a gooseberry!

Grainne doesn't tell us about the actual living arrangements between herself and her siblings, and whether the dream of living in a tiny flat is an actual or metaphoric reflection of her situation. In any case, the dream paints a clear picture of the status of the relationships between the siblings, which is too close and bordering on incestuous. So boundaries have to be put in place.

This is Grainne's dream, and it needn't be brought to the attention of her brothers and their girlfriends. She needs to take this dream seriously, and take steps to distance herself from what's going on. The adjective 'chaotic', which means great confusion, originally referred to a chasm or abyss. 'Uncomfortable', which means not enjoyable or consoling, derives from the Latin '*confortare*', to strengthen, which indicates hope. Grainne should apply all of those meanings to herself and live them out, in order to stop the confusion and extricate herself in a determined manner from the emotional gulf into which the dream is showing her that she has sunk.

Hannah's dream of having an affair with her best friend

✦ ✧ ✦ ✧ ✦

I keep dreaming that I'm having an affair with my best friend. I'm a married woman and my best friend is male. – Hannah

✦ ✧ ✦ ✧ ✦

What an interesting dream for Hannah, and as she says, it's one she 'keeps dreaming'. This means it hasn't been fully understood nor acted upon, which is why it repeats. Or maybe it repeats because she enjoys it so much!

The first question to ask is whether she is indeed having an affair with her best friend. Or is she doing anything with her best friend that could be construed as having an affair? For example, spending too much time with him – time that should be spent with her husband. The dream continually brings to her attention the fact that she is having an affair. So maybe it's a worry of Hannah's, or a fear, or, as Freud would suggest, a wish to have an affair with her best friend. As a first step, it would be important to unravel the truth here.

On a metaphorical level, the dream is registering a deep and intimate connection between Hannah and this man. So I'd ask her to define what qualities he has that she finds so attractive. Is it his intelligence or his strength, or that he has a beautiful nature, or an attractive body?

The qualities that she sees in her best friend in the dream are actually her own qualities. Having projected them outwards onto her best friend, she needs to take them back and own them properly. They belong to her, although her friend obviously has a hook on which she is able to hang these qualities.

I draw this interpretation because in the dream Hannah has an affair with this man – in other words, she is intimately connected with his qualities, with what he represents, and she needs to make sure that she incarnates the masculine qualities that she sees and admires in her best friend in her own life as a married woman in order to become a more balanced individual. That's the internal work that Hannah needs to do here.

The dream doesn't infer that Hannah should have an affair with her best friend, which, as a married woman, inevitably would cause too many people too much hurt and pain. But I note that her best friend is not her husband. If she's not in love with her husband, and also wants to end the marriage, then she needs to face that situation honestly. They got married, so at one time there was affection between them. Hannah owes it to her husband, and the life that they shared together, to disentangle the situation properly before moving on with her life, and embracing whatever the future holds for her with someone else. At the moment her unconscious already knows the truth, and it needs her to take that new information from the dream on board. So if Hannah faces the truth head on, it will set her free.

Irene's dream of falling in love with a man who keeps getting taken away

✦ ✧ ✦ ✧ ✦

I keep dreaming of falling in love with a man and he keeps getting taken away from me by big gangs of men. I wake up crying. I can see his face but I don't recognize him. Can you dream about people you have never seen in your life? – Irene

✦ ✧ ✦ ✧ ✦

*D*oesn't that opening sentence of Irene's dream say it all? She says, 'I keep dreaming of falling in love with a man, and he keeps getting taken away from me'. There's almost a child-like quality in that complaint: as soon as she gets something, it's taken away from her. And there's a further interesting piece of information here. Irene says of the man she falls in love with, 'he keeps getting taken away from me by big gangs of men'. In other words, it's 'the lads' that take him away, or he's too caught up in the lads, or 'big gangs of men', as she phrases it.

As 'a big gang of men' is a collective, the dream could be pointing towards a problem on the collective level of the unconscious, which prevents Irene from continuing a relationship with the man she loves. We have to go back a generation to get to that collective level: Irene may be too much caught up with her father, or over-identified with her father, who keeps getting taken away from her by her mother, and that difficulty could be preventing her from falling in love with another man.

Irene says, 'I can see his face, but I don't recognise him.' What do we hear in that? To 'recognise' means to acknowledge, and she's not acknowledging something that's staring her in the face. It can also mean to treat as valid, so Irene is saying that she's not treating the man she falls in love with as being valid, which doesn't bode well for sustaining a relationship. I'd ask Irene, who does that face remind you of? Whose does it resemble? What can you say about it? How would you describe it? Those answers will give her a good indication of what's robbing her of her enjoyment.

Irene says, 'I wake up crying,' meaning wailing, or making a noise of grief or pain. Originally the word 'crying' meant begging or imploring, which is a cry for help, a need that should be responded to. And Irene finishes with a question, 'Can you dream about people you've never seen in your life?' The answer is yes, but she must remember that it's her dream. Irene has chosen the actors to represent something that's relevant to her, so the people she has never seen in her life represent a part of herself of which she has been unconscious up to now. She needs to know about these aspects of herself, and to acknowledge them, so that she can make better choices in her life going forward. Thus equipped, Irene will be able to steer herself onto a better course, so that she can choose men who will no longer be taken away from her.

Niamh's dream of jogging with a colleague

✦ ✧ ✦ ✧ ✦

I dreamt that I was jogging through a forest with a colleague. He was boasting that he could run two kilometres in a minute! We passed an abandoned house, and he said that he saw an old man in it looking out at us. The house changed the whole feeling of the dream, and made it creepy and scary. – Niamh

✦ ✧ ✦ ✧ ✦

This dream is about the 'look', which is uncanny really, because we're not able to truthfully read a person's look unless they tell us what it is about. An unfathomable look can also reduce us to shame. Here in Niamh's dream, it's an old man's look.

Let's start at the beginning. Niamh goes for a gentle run with a male colleague, who boasts he can run two kilometres in a minute, so in her dream he's showing off to her that he's fit and healthy – suitable partner material. Jogging brings with it the undercurrent of horizontal jogging, which is slang for sexual intercourse, and there's always a sexual aspect to a dream.

Niamh then links herself and her colleague through using the first person plural 'we' by saying 'we passed an abandoned house'. This abandoned house represents the past: it's likely that it once housed a family who have passed on. Niamh's colleague says that 'he saw an old man in it looking out at us', underlining the masculine perspective. The old man is a verbal stand-in for the father, and as Niamh says, 'The house changed the whole feeling of the dream, and made it creepy and scary.' So Niamh reads the look from the old man transposed onto a house from the past as one of disapproval, which changed the whole feeling of the dream, making it 'creepy and scary'. The word 'creepy' means having a feeling of horror. In American English it means despicable, and originally referred to a robber or sneak thief. So Niamh's enjoyment of jogging with her colleague has been robbed from her by a feeling of contempt.

The house is a general indicator of where we live, and figuratively, of the attitudes that we have. Since the house is abandoned, these are outworn attitudes of censure and disapproval that are coming from an earlier time in Niamh's life, and they belong to the old man. Niamh needs to assign them clearly to the place where they belong, and site them firmly in the past in order to bring her real attitudes up to date.

So the dream paints Niamh this picture to show her that she should enjoy jogging with this male colleague. It is telling her to live her life to the full, without suffering the unwanted shame from her past.

6

Journey Dreams

*J*ourney dreams refer to both inner and outer aspects of the personality. The hero's journey in dreams is a representation of the various psychological stages we have to go through in order to become mature human beings. Often the drama of the dream can point out obstacles on the way that we need to deal with before we can move on to the next stage. Neurotic conflicts result in the shirking of appropriate life tasks, and journey dreams highlight these impediments.

There are often three aspects to the journey: the preparation or departure, with its emotional mix of separation, anxiety and excitement; the journey itself, with its various setbacks and triumphs; and finally the joyful return, with its achievements resulting in a tangible redemption. These rites of passage today are most often seen in the travel associated with the gap year, or the university study abroad programme. While our culture may not recognise the sacred nature of these journeys, they're grounded in the age-old mythical patterns of the unconscious, and designed to transform our lives.

The journey motif in dreams dramatises the possibility of change, especially when the person moves from one place to another. A night sea journey from west to east is a common motif, and symbolises the transit of the sun from sunset to dawn. The hero goes underground into darkness, which represents death. The journey is a spiritual pilgrimage in which the dreamer becomes acquainted with the nature of death – a journey of release, renunciation and atonement in a spirit of compassion, and then comes back to the surface – or resurrects, if you like – to bring back to the community the wisdom gained from such a major, transformative change.

Finn's dream of winning a radio competition

I had a strange dream last night where I won a radio competition and, strangely, Ryan Tubridy arrived at my college! Strange and all, but Ryan then stayed at my house, and the next day we embarked on a journey to somewhere that I didn't know. The dream ended and I was completely confused. – Finn

I think Finn's dream is really complimentary about the Irish broadcaster Ryan Tubridy! In the dream, Finn won a radio competition. You can read that in two ways: that Finn won a competition featured on the radio, or that he won a competition to be on the radio.

Who arrives at his college but Ryan Tubridy. It's in this public learning institution that Ryan is introduced in the dream. The dream then moves on to a private level, where Ryan stays in his house, the place where Finn lives: here Ryan is inhabiting Finn's personal space.

The movement in the dream is from night to day: 'I had a strange dream last night … and the next day we embarked on a journey to somewhere that I didn't know'. The word 'embark' means to go on board a ship, so the trip to be undertaken by both Finn and Ryan is the metaphorical night sea journey to do with psychological growth, where at some level Finn is required in this dream to learn to communicate through speech alone, because a radio transmits voice signals without the distraction of any visual cues. The word 'competition' means to strive against others. We're all born into the sea of language, and our task is to elbow others out of the way, and to make that communal legacy our own, to turn speech into a tool with which to communicate our inmost self to others and, in the process, develop ourselves creatively.

The dream suggests that Finn has achieved this as he says, 'I won a radio competition'. Ryan, as a radio personality, is obviously in the position of a teacher, guide or guru for Finn on this journey. Ryan can fulfil the promise of the radio competition for him, and take him on a radio journey, which is a very particular journey where speech is privileged, and where Finn is a winner. What a lovely, lovely dream.

And what should we make of the word 'strange' that Finn uses frequently throughout his dream? The etymology of the word means foreign, unknown, unfamiliar and alien, so by peppering his dream with the word 'strange', Finn emphasises that he's completely outside his comfort zone by embarking on a journey with Ryan 'to somewhere that I didn't know'. Even though Ryan is a Shadow figure embodying traits and capacities that apparently have never been used before, Finn also acknowledges that Ryan, the radio personality, is an expert on radio, so he is in good hands and can trust him.

Finn's unconscious is clearly suggesting that he has the ability to become a broadcaster or at least to ground himself in speech. He says, 'The dream ended and I was completely confused.' He uses 'confused' in the sense of confounded and mixed up, which relates to the word 'strange' that he used earlier in the dream. Finn has been thrown into disorder by this dream, and yet it needs to be honoured in some way, and not 'ended' lest Finn end up defeated and frustrated, which was the original meaning of the word confused. Strange indeed!

The question Finn now needs to ask himself and – more importantly – to respond to is: how is he going to incarnate the spirit of his dream? Is he going to become a broadcaster? And if not, how can Finn make the best use of use his voice to progress the oneiric metaphor of winning a radio competition?

Rachel's dream about going on holidays

✦ ✧ ✦ ✧ ✦

I keep dreaming about going on holidays, but to different destinations each time. I only ever dream about packing and going on the plane, never arriving at my destination. I've had this dream about seven times. – Rachel

✦ ✧ ✦ ✧ ✦

The way that Rachel presents this dream is worth paying attention to. She says, 'I keep dreaming about going on holidays'. So Rachel's unconscious keeps compensating for the humdrum, boring responsibilities in her everyday life, helping her to escape from these by literally taking flight while she's sleeping.

Rachel says, 'I only ever dream about packing and going on the plane, never arriving'. So there's the preparatory departure phase involved, and the journeying of 'going on the plane'. This can also be part of the holiday, but her dreams do not include the actual arrival at the interchangable destinations. Isn't that a great metaphor? Rachel's unconscious is pointing out to her that it's the journey, and not the different destinations, that is important!

I'm reading 'going on the plane' as the journey, but Rachel could mean boarding the plane, in which case the journey is absent. And in the unconscious, an absence is the same as a presence: it is consciousness which introduces that binary opposition. Both meanings have Rachel referring to the journey, in any case.

Finally Rachel says, 'I've had this dream about seven times'. Now seven is a mystical or sacred number, which from time immemorial has meant completion or perfection. There are seven days in creation, seven days in the week, seven virtues, seven ages of man according to Shakespeare, seven corporal works of mercy, seven gifts of the Holy Spirit, and seven heavens in Islam. So seven is a very special, lucky number.

This is an important dream for Rachel. If she lives out the fact that it's the journey that is important and not the arrival at the destination, she'll be very lucky indeed. In other words, she will learn far more from what she puts into the journey of life, rather than striving for a particular result. If there's a destination as a result of her efforts, then that's an added bonus. But there doesn't have to be a destination, because it's how she prepares for the journey of life that's important, seeking her reward within the journey itself.

If Rachel follows that programme that her unconscious is proposing – preparing for and embarking on that journey – it will bring Rachel untold spiritual wealth, and she'll be in seventh heaven!

Helen's dream of being a cowboy

✦ ✧ ✦ ✧ ✦

I dreamt last night that I was a cowboy. I was riding a horse over the desert and had to destroy a statue and I would be rich. The statue turned out to be a statue of my best friend. In the dream, I woke up although I was still asleep, and was in a tranquil spa! It was lovely! – Helen

✦ ✧ ✦ ✧ ✦

*I*sn't that a lovely dream to do with going on a personal journey and finding treasure? It's a version of the Greek myth 'Jason and the Golden Fleece', in which Helen has to accomplish tasks in order to become a whole human being.

In the dream, Helen is a cowboy, riding a horse over the desert. What do we think that makes her? Independent, adventurous, exploring, self-sufficient, tough, heroic – the best of the archetypal masculine qualities. The terrain in which Helen is operating is desert, a barren region that is inhospitable to man. So at some level Helen is very much on her own; indeed, the word 'desert' comes from the Latin '*desertum*', literally a thing abandoned. So whatever is going on in Helen's life, her unconscious registers being forsaken: Helen is lonely, all by herself. I wonder if this loneliness is due to her best friend being emotionally cold, like a statue, or if it is saying that the masculine qualities of being a cowboy leave Helen herself diminished, as if she has abandoned herself.

She dreamt she was a cowboy. The original meaning of the word 'boy' was a male child or servant. It's also possibly borrowing from the Old French, meaning fettered or shackled. So there's an indication in the language Helen uses that she doesn't have her freedom.

Helen's psychological task in the dream is to destroy the statue, and if she accomplishes this, she'll be rich. Most statues are made on commission to commemorate an influential person, but the statue Helen has to destroy is a statue of her best friend, which seems to suggest that Helen is over-valuing this friend, to the extent that the dream requires her to become an iconoclast, and destroy the statue of this venerated person, her 'best' friend. This is Helen's task and, according to the dream, this refashioning will result in riches, which means that in her case, Helen's personality will benefit from cutting her best friend down to size.

In conclusion she says, 'In the dream I woke up ... and was in a tranquil spa. It was lovely.' By paying attention to the life lesson in the dream and destroying the statue of her friend, a destruction that on the face of it might appear violent but which needs the masculine qualities of the cowboy to complete the task, Helen wakes up. This awakening leaves her in a health and beauty spa. A spa is quite a calm and feminine space for Helen to wake up in! Fully inhabiting her femininity is the riches that this dream offers to her. Helen's reaction is 'It was lovely.' In Germanic as in Celtic, the old Indo-European word for love assumed the meaning 'free'. So the fettered or shackled boy at the beginning of this dream has turned into a free woman at the end: quite a transformative journey indeed that Helen's unconscious has mapped out for her in this dream!

Gareth's dream of being in a wheelchair

✦ ✧ ✦ ✧ ✦

I had a dream that I was in a wheelchair but I was able to walk because whenever I got to stairs, I was able to walk up. I walked into a cathedral-like room where three girls were talking. A voice yelled that I was not allowed to be there. The room darkened and I was pushed from the room. Outside there were people wearing white and gold who were fighting. Then I suddenly woke up! – Gareth

✦ ✧ ✦ ✧ ✦

The first line of a dream is very important, because it sets the scene. To help us interpret it, often it's useful to add the words 'and this is my life' to the end of the first line. Gareth says, 'I had a dream that I was in a wheelchair … [and this is my life!]'. So we can understand that the opening line is saying that Gareth is an invalid – a sickly person, weak or disabled through illness or injury. Interestingly, the word was originally pronounced 'in-*val*-id' meaning not valid. And Gareth goes on to say, 'I was able to walk'. So there's a pun or a joke about what's valid and what's not valid at the beginning of Gareth's dream, an ambivalence or a contradiction that sets the scene: there's a definite doubt hanging over Gareth being able, or valid.

The next scene took place in a cathedral-like room, where three girls were talking. A voice yelled that Gareth was not allowed to be there, and he was pushed from the room after it darkened and went into a shadow. The cathedral space is feminine, womb- or cave-like, and archetypally three girls represent the three ages of the feminine: the maiden, the married woman, and the crone. So this is definitely female territory that Gareth has intruded upon, and the voice yells out to him that he's not allowed to be there, because he's male; it's not valid for a man to be intruding upon what is a woman's space. It's appropriate that it should draw on the Shadow because, of necessity, a man's feminine side is not as developed as his masculinity. Once again, and for a second time, the dream is painting a picture that Gareth needs to take up his masculine position.

The final scene, which suddenly wakes up Gareth, takes place outside where 'people wearing white and gold' were fighting. These colours are actually opposites. In alchemical terms the white is known as *albedo*, which is the white light of the moon, the world of the unconscious where everything is changeable, full of fantasy, quiet and introverted, and which is also regarded as a feminine space. The gold is known as *rubedo*, which is the golden world of the sun, order, consciousness, fiery and extraverted, traditionally masculine.

So to conclude, Gareth's journey dream is marking a transition, where Gareth is forging a path for himself as a man, where he's questioning how to be valid in the world and how to be a real man, and whether he should be introverted or extraverted. There's a fight going on between his feminine side and his nascent masculinity. Gareth feels he's not able, but the dream asks him not to be deceived by that: it assures him that he is able, and that he'll be able to climb the stairs and take the necessary steps to become the person that he should be. It's a wonderfully encouraging and transformative dream for Gareth. It's now time for him to put these lessons from his dream into practice!

Jeanine's dream of climbing into the sky

✦ ◇ ✦ ◇ ✦

I have a recurring dream where I find a rope hanging from the sky. I climb the rope into the sky, higher and higher until I'm climbing through clouds. When I reach the top, there's a circular platform with a well in the middle. There's a girl whose face is blurry. I lean over and look into the well, but before I see my reflection the dream ends. – Jeanine

✦ ◇ ✦ ◇ ✦

The drama of Jeanine's journey dream shows us that Jeanine is inclined to get too high, too manic, as she says, 'I climb a rope into the sky, higher and higher until I'm climbing through clouds.' And when she gets to her destination, she looks into a well. Jeanine says that the dream ends before she's able to see her reflection, but she also says that 'there's a girl whose face is blurry', which is obviously a transposition of her own reflection in the water. So by going too high, Jeanine ends up looking at her reflection, which she doesn't recognise as being herself. And she says, 'before I see my reflection the dream ends', which doubly underlines that's there's a problem to do with seeing her reflection.

It's the mother who shapes our perception of ourselves. We won't feel that we're desirable unless we've experienced a time in our very early life when we knew we were the apple of our mother's eye. This also presupposes that the very young child realises at some later time that it's conceivable this might not happen. This is an anxiety that can haunt a child, and cause it to go on a journey to achieve this, like climbing a phallic-like object hanging down from the sky.

In classical mythology, the sky belongs to Zeus, god the father. So by identifying with her father's realm, Jeanine hopes to achieve the recognition that her father holds in her mother's affection. Her journey as illustrated in the dream now becomes a life-long quest to capture her mother's attention.

Jeanine's dream draws on two motifs of myth and fairy tale – the rope into the sky, and the well. Both of these motifs have been refined in the telling down through the ages, and offer wisdom. In the mythical tale about Jack and the Beanstalk, which is found in differing forms among many peoples, Jack sells his cow for magic beans, and when his mother gives out to him, he throws the beans in the garden, and overnight they grow into an almighty stalk, which he climbs up into the sky and eventually finds a pot of gold that he brings back to his mother. The second myth Jeanine's dream employs comes from Greece. Narcissus was a beautiful youth who mistook his reflection in a fountain for somebody else. He repeatedly tried to reach this unrecognised person, but he couldn't, so he pined away until his death. This illustrates a potential warning to Jeanine that by staying stuck at such an early transition stage on her life's journey, she risks the death of wasting away with desire and yearning.

As human beings we're not meant to climb into the sky other than in an aeroplane, and Jeanine says she was going 'higher and higher until I'm climbing through clouds'. Whether these are clouds of marijuana smoke that cause Jeanine to get high she doesn't say! And like the failed effort made by Narcissus, Jeanine says, 'I lean over and look into the well, but before I see my reflection the dream ends.' Jeanine loses sight of herself because the dream offered by her unconscious ends. The dream leaves her waking, conscious self to realise its conclusion; there isn't a prescribed outcome. Jeanine is meant to wake up to this dangerous situation. The dream also tells Jeanine that as things stand, she's left looking into nothingness, oblivion. Perhaps her mother didn't love her, or maybe she died before Jeanine had a chance to experience properly being the apple of her eye.

She begins by saying that this is 'a recurring dream', so its message has not been received nor understood, hence the repetition urging her to move on from constantly seeking her mother's love, and to keep her feet planted firmly on the ground. Interestingly, the word 'rope' originally meant a shoelace, so 'I find a rope hanging from the sky' is a doubly inappropriate image since it's out of place here.

When Jeanine gets high, she doesn't recognise herself and others, which has narcissistic echoes of being self-absorbed. Jeanine is having the dream to warn her about this, so that she doesn't become too haughty and look down on other people. The dream urges Jeanine to remain humble enough to make relationship connections with people other than herself through being grounded, and to move on from that very early relationship with her mother.

Jeanine can bring some balance to bear on this situation. If she stays at the centre of the see-saw of life, then she won't swing too high up into the clouds!

Fiona's dream of Sydney

✦ ✧ ✦ ✧ ✦

Last night I had a déjà vu dream. I dreamt that I was in Sydney. I went to a shopping centre and walked around some old streets and saw a pier. In my dream I knew I had been to all these places before. When I woke up I realised I hadn't been to these places before in real life, but I had been there in another dream. – Fiona

✦ ✧ ✦ ✧ ✦

So this is the second dream that Fiona has had about being in Sydney. Fiona doesn't tell us what Sydney means to her, but her personal associations with Sydney could point us towards what this dream is getting at. Sydney obviously holds something special for Fiona, because the dream is repeating in her unconscious. This time she has remembered to submit it for analysis, and that act of honouring of her dream has brought back the memory of the first dream. She also acknowledges her experience of the first dream within her second dream, so it is a dream within a dream.

We can think about what Sydney could represent. It's the other side of the world, as far away from Europe as it's possible to get. To that extent, it's representative of the unconscious, of the other side of consciousness. Fiona immerses herself in this other side, and allows the unconscious to have its say in her life.

Sydney is also representative of the outdoor Australian way of life and extraversion, which could be a way of compensating for the introverted parts of Fiona's personality, and the internal way that she lives her life in Ireland. Sydney is also regarded as the cultural centre of Australia, famous for its opera house, so it's representative of creativity, particularly through using the human voice to express feeling.

Making choices, appreciating the past as well as the new, and being open to the outside world and unknown experiences can take Fiona out of her narrow perspectives. On emotional and spiritual levels, these are all possibilities expressed through the contextual web of associations with the creative drama of Fiona's dream.

She says, 'I went to a shopping centre and walked around some old streets and saw a pier. In my dream I knew I had been to all these places before.' These are everyday activities that could be done here at home. However, a lot of young adventurers go to Sydney in their gap year. It provides a broadening of experience that stays with them for the rest of their lives, and which is of enormous benefit, enriching their personalities. It teaches them how to manage their new-found independence, and shows them that they have the ability to survive and thrive in the world of adulthood.

Fiona says, 'I had a déjà vu dream. I dreamt that I was in Sydney … When I woke up I realized that I hadn't been to these places before in real life, but had been there in another dream.' So the awakening related to the dream raises a question about the correct framework with which to view this. The stage on which this drama is performed moves to another, previous one, which also references the revisionary nature of the personal journey that Fiona has undertaken, and has experienced in her dream. The return, or awakening, refers to a different dream, the very first one she had about Sydney.

Freud always made a distinction between the manifest, disguised content of the dream, which is what Fiona relates, and the undisguised latent content, which Freud says is what the dream is about. Here the latent content turns out to be the previous first dream. So Fiona is having a dream of a dream. Listen carefully to what she says: 'When I woke up' – this awakening is what is important – 'I realised I hadn't been to these places before in real life' – Fiona recognises the lack in her life – 'but I had been there in another dream.' In the latent content of the dream, Fiona is saying that it's her dream to go to Sydney.

Fiona's déjà vu dream is grounding her in familiarity while she's experiencing the challenge of the new: the phrase 'déjà vu' means to perceive a new situation as if it had occurred before.

In other words, while Fiona is asleep, she re-visits areas of experience to update her strategies for survival. This is one of the functions of the dream: it helps us to consolidate our strengths, in order to better deal with what's going to be presented to us in the days to come.

Fiona needs to follow her idea of bliss and undertake that journey to Sydney. Whatever it holds for her, her unconscious is saying that she needs to experience Sydney in real life. This is what Fiona's déjà vu dream is teaching her.

Ita's dream of getting lost

✦ ✧ ✦ ✧ ✦

I was riding a bike from college. I got lost and ended up at a friend's house, who was making robots that looked like humans! It was weird, but funny. There were these robot people hanging up all over the place, like at a butcher's. We were laughing in the dream. – Ita

✦ ✧ ✦ ✧ ✦

*I*ta says that she was riding a bike, which is a very individual thing to do. It's not like driving a car, which can be collective because we can share the ride with several people. So we know Ita is on her individual journey after leaving college. But she gets lost, which can be an unnerving experience, particularly if it recalls terrifying memories we all have from childhood in which we got lost in a supermarket or at a shopping centre. However, Ita ends up at a friend's house, which is very comforting because she has support; she's no longer isolated nor on her own.

Now comes the odd detail, which is very specific, and which Ita finds 'weird, but funny': her friend was making robots that looked like humans. And these robot people were hanging up all over the place, like at a butcher's, presumably like the carcasses of animals hanging on meat hooks. There's something unsettling about these images in the dream, even if Ita thought they were funny. I think the dream is bringing to Ita's attention in graphic form something about her friend that she has either overlooked, or never saw as plainly before. The dream is very clear about this: Ita's friend makes robots that look like humans, and she has them 'hanging up all over the place', like the dead meat in a butcher's shop.

A robot is a mechanical device that does some of the work of a human being. It derives from the Czech word '*robota*', meaning work or labour, which is related to the Slavic word for slave. So the dream is saying that her friend makes slaves that look like humans. In the dream, Ita finds this 'weird but funny'.

The word 'weird' means having the power to control the fate of men. It's a trickster motif in the dream. It is apparently 'funny', as Ita says, but originally the word 'fun' referred to a jester, and meant to trick, hoax or joke in the sense of cheating or cajoling people. It tells us that it's not to be taken at face value. There's a real truth lurking under the surface here about Ita's friend, perhaps about the way that her friend relates to and controls other people: he or she somehow demeans them, turning them into working objects, something you would see on a meat-rack in a butcher's. That's what this dream is saying.

So Ita should be careful. She is a bright girl coming from college, but the dream points out that she has lost her way.

Ita should also watch her step with this friend, because she doesn't want to end up as a trophy on a wall!

7

Trickster and Shapeshifter Dreams

*T*rickster and Shapeshifter dreams correspond to the earliest, least developed period of life. The Trickster has the mentality of an infant, who is concerned with the gratification of his primary needs. He has a low level of intelligence, and he can manifest as cruel, unfeeling and cynical because of his animal nature.

The Trickster or Shapeshifter passes from one mischievous deed to another, playing tricks on us, such as initiating slips of the tongue, causing us to mishear something, getting us to lose or forget things at the least opportune times, or creating mindless absurdities and unnecessary disasters for us. He's like a collective version of the Shadow, having all of the unrecognised or ignored traits of our culture. He can surface in the mob mentality of the masses, so that the Trickster or Shapeshifter is potentially extremely dangerous. He constantly reminds us that our civilisation was built upon our animal nature, and that we need to pay the closest attention to that fact.

In mythology the god Hermes/Mercury is the Trickster par excellence, and his statue is atop the General Post Office in Dublin, because he is the messenger of the gods. He is also the god of crossroads, of windfalls, and he leads souls to and from the underworld. In Ancient Greek mythology, the phallus of Hermes penetrates from the known into the unknown world, so he oversees aspects of sexuality as well.

The Trickster motif has been written about in the myth cycles and folk tales of all peoples, overturning the established order and reducing the world around him to chaos and pandemonium. He was always seen in clowns, fools, jesters, satyrs and devils, and at carnivals, circuses and funfairs. This means that he still has a function in our lives today.

On a positive note, the Trickster or Shapeshifter reminds us that it's always possible for a situation that appears intractable to turn around. This process is known as enantiodromia, and stems from a Greek word that means running in contrary ways. It refers not only to the process by which something becomes its opposite, but also the arresting effects of this. In this way, the Trickster or Shapeshifter has the potential to initiate the most profound transformation, even though the change itself could be painful.

Sarah's dream of her tutor being a transgender serial killer

✦ ✧ ✦ ✧ ✦

I dreamt last night that one of my college tutors told us she was a serial killer, and that she was a transgender person. She did it not because of gender identity, but as a disguise to escape from the police. Then he made fun of my weight. – Sarah

✦ ✧ ✦ ✧ ✦

Sarah's college tutor appears in her dream as a serial killer. That's a very dangerous figure, so we can surmise that Sarah feels very threatened by this tutor, or by something about her.

Furthermore, the serial killer is a male-to-female transgender person: a Shapeshifter. Although the tutor presents as female, she has crossed gender identity, and Sarah is able to detect that behind this female is a man. In other words, the tutor has the archetypal masculine qualities of the alpha male – tough, strong and forceful – together with the attributes of the Shapeshifter – cruelty, a lack of empathy and cynicism.

The reason for this cross-gender disguise, according to Sarah's dream, is, 'to escape from the police', from the enforcers of the law. So this tutor is lawless to the extent that she/he is not bound by a law that applies to everyone else: a Trickster indeed. Often a person's father can come up in a dream in those terms, so I wonder if difficulties with Sarah's father are the motor behind this particular drama.

'Then he made fun of my weight.' Comments about weight can be a very touchy subject and can hurt another person. We're aware of this today, and we would never normally refer to someone's weight, so another boundary is being crossed here. And this is the first time that Sarah refers to her tutor as 'he'.

The dream draws attention to murderous impulses through a variety of devices – a serial killer, not being bound by the law, breaching of boundaries that leads to confusion over sexual identity, and to saying things that you wouldn't normally say. So while the dream shows real fear of the tutor, maybe even of Sarah's father in the present or in the past, it's also referencing other subjects that have a more personal resonance for Sarah under the rubric of the Lord of Misrule. This figure, associated with the Elizabethan period but whose lineage goes back to the Saturnalia festival of Roman times, presided over a period of licensed anarchy where convention was overturned: commoners became kings, men dressed as women, and masters waited on their servants.

Since our dreams present aspects of ourselve that we might have difficulty recognising, much less assimilating, the gender confusion in this dream reflects a problem with which Sarah is grappling. The fact that she turns this transgender person into a serial killer shows the depth of her horrified reaction to such a situation.

It could be important for Sarah to go and talk about these topics with someone, particularly as the dream comes up in such a threatening form. I use that word 'topics' deliberately here, meaning matter to be treated in speech, because it was first recorded by the eminent Irish writer Jonathan Swift. Originally it meant to tolerate, allow, agree to and make available, which is why it could be healthy for Sarah to spend time considering the many topics that are being articulated in this dream from every perspective, and see whether what they bring to Sarah's attention can – even in some small way – be incorporated into her wider outlook. That way they will be less threatening and more manageable.

The Shapeshifter motif to do with gender in this dream means that Sarah can be persuaded or, given the underlying motif, is more likely to be tricked into embracing the whole of her better self, despite the frightening Shadow qualities expressed in this dream. And such an outlook is really hopeful and transformative. But she should also be careful.

Kevin's dream of a roller coaster, Superman and an octopus

◆ ◇ ◆ ◇ ◆

I dreamt that I climbed on top of a roller coaster to find my sister with Superman and an octopus. The octopus then picked me up and threw me off, and the dream ended. – Kevin

◆ ◇ ◆ ◇ ◆

This is a Trickster dream. The archetype of the Trickster is embodied in jesters, clowns, scapegoats, devils and the Greek god Pan. In medieval carnivals the Trickster presided over a reversal of the order that we expect, and he also continues to manifest many other images of folly. The Trickster causes chaos, and a Trickster dream tricks us into recognising the truth.

The main image here is of a roller coaster, a typical carnival image. And in the dream, Kevin is joined by the comic book and movie hero Superman – who is all powerful and can fly through the air – and an octopus, which is a highly intelligent, very flexible and fluid animal, which can fly through water, and can change colour. Both of these are typical Trickster and Shapeshifter motifs. The symbol of the octopus can also refer to an organised power with far-reaching influence, especially when harmful or destructive.

The Trickster, by playing tricks, points to a potential disaster. Here in Kevin's dream he says, 'The octopus picked me up and threw me off [the top of the roller coaster]'. But in this Trickster fantasy world Superman is also there, and he can save Kevin.

However, the Trickster and Shapeshifter dream serves to astonish and awaken us. It asks questions of us, and it won't allow them to be ignored, so the first step is to find solutions and answers to problems.

In the dream, Kevin says, 'I climbed to the top of a roller coaster to find my sister'. This is a ridiculous and dangerous effort to be making; it's literally way over the top. What does a roller coaster suggest as a metaphor? It represents emotional highs and lows, thrills and terror. So the dream is showing Kevin that he's literally on a roller coaster! Kevin is accompanied by Superman, who helps people in difficult situations, and by an animal that also helps the hero, an octopus. However, here the octopus picked him up and threw him off the roller coaster, which is a disaster that paradoxically leads to the correct conclusion – the ending of the dream Kevin has of being his sister's protector.

This roller coaster dream tricks Kevin into the truth that his sister doesn't need to be looked out for or minded. Kevin needs to change his attitude towards her, and just make normal efforts to remain in touch. No matter what Kevin's situation in life, if he finds he is making superhuman efforts, there's something wrong, and he needs to take stock. Certainly, as a first step, he should embrace being thrown off this particular roller coaster, otherwise the Trickster or Shapeshifter, which are universal patterns in the unconscious, will make it happen in his relationship with his sister, and the result will be much more dangerous, even fatal. So he should stay off the roller coaster, and not involve himself in his sister's dramas. She can find herself.

8
Nightmares

nightmare is an evil, female spirit who afflicts sleepers with a feeling of suffocation. The Anglo-Saxon word '*mare*' refers to a demon or goblin, and its predecessor, the Sanskrit word '*mara*', refers to a destructive force or destroyer, which in turn may come from '*mar*', to crush. The common features induced by nightmares are intense dread, paralysis of movement, and a sensation of crushing upon the chest, which interferes with breathing.

A nightmare is an anxiety dream in which the feelings of fear and terror are experienced to such an intense degree that the dreamer is overwhelmed and often is forced into wakefulness. There's an overpowering sense of danger in a nightmare. The dreamer is under threat of a violent attack from aggression, castration, separation, abandonment, being devoured, or even from losing his identity. Regression to an intense state of infantile helplessness in the face of such overwhelming anxiety is a very common feature.

In nightmares, a threatening situation in current life can often become linked with the memory of traumatic childhood incidents. The life and death struggle that's presented in the nightmare is represented in terms that are typical of early childhood conflicts: little people threatened by giants, for example.

Night terrors are characteristic of very young children. Those who experience parental hostility, ongoing hatred, or repeated destructive threats to their welfare from adults or siblings are particularly prone to nightmares. Parental fears that are transmitted or communicated to young people who have no capacity to deal with them also result in nightmares. Being over-protected by smothering parents who are too present can trigger nightmares as well.

Most children encounter environments that they perceive as threatening, in which they can feel helpless. The deepest anxieties caused by nightmares are found in children before the age of five, when the ability to differentiate between the outside and the inside is in a fluid state, and is just developing. Young children explore the world with their mouths, and aggressive, devouring figures are prominent in children's nightmares – both being eaten up and devouring another person and then feeling the other person inside are common. As adults, we have an ongoing problem with the opposition between inside and outside, which, as our dreams disclose, are not discrete categories, but continuous with each other. The capacity to maintain the distinction between a dream and reality is fought for from babyhood through childhood onwards, so it is also subject to disruption and regression in adult life. The after effects of a bad dream can linger throughout the day and trouble us.

We tend also to link external threats to our own unacceptable wishes, and to project these drives and impulses onto our dreams' hallucinatory images. We respond to these images as if they were real monsters or threatening events. So raging figures can not only represent our parents and parental figures, but in our nightmares they're infused with our own aggressive impulses and desires as well, wishes we'd normally keep under wraps.

Major anxieties are generated in the course of a person's psychosexual development. Because of the regressive aspect of nightmares, a very early and distorted conception of sexuality is often revived and given lurid expression in our dreams.

Nightmares are concerned with matters of life and death, so they should be taken very seriously indeed. They're designed to get our attention in as forceful a way as possible, so that we can keep our wits about us, and take some action to ward off a potential imminent destruction. While nightmares can sometimes indicate an imbalance in our personalities, or a disturbed integration of various aspects of our personalities, generally these severe anxiety dreams occur at times of important change in our lives. They herald the beginning of significant undertakings that take us out of our comfort zones, or mark critical shifts in the psychological development of our personalities that can work towards our good if we consciously choose to take on board what our nightmares are telling us.

Eamonn's dream of a betting shop

✦ ✧ ✦ ✧ ✦

I dreamt that night that I was in a betting shop. I kept winning and was really happy and sweating with excitement! Everyone was cheering me on. Then it turned nasty. People got aggressive with me and I had to try and escape or be injured. I woke up in a state. – Eamonn

✦ ✧ ✦ ✧ ✦

This dream shows Eamonn's ambivalence about betting, the trickster motif of a windfall. It displays in dramatic form the emotional conflict he's experiencing – as he says, 'I woke up in a state!' On the one hand, Eamonn says, 'I kept winning and was really happy and sweating with excitement. Everyone was cheering me on.' And on the other hand he says, if Eamonn were to remain in the betting shop, he'd be injured, so he has to try and escape. The word 'escape' literally means to get out of one's cape, to leave a pursuer with just one's cape, to get away by the skin of your teeth, or to barely make it to safety. The bottom line in Eamonn's warning dream is very clear.

Eamonn uses the strong phrase 'sweating with excitement' to describe himself when he was winning. It suggests a level of excitement that's above the ordinary – a euphoric recall, if you like, or a real turn-on. However, 'Then it turned nasty.' In the dream, his betting activity tips over into its opposite. For a gambler, this would mean that he starts losing, which Eamonn doesn't mention; rather, the nastiness he talks about is displaced onto people's aggression towards him. The reversal of fortune from winning to turning nasty invites aggression towards him, which illustrates the Trickster or Shapeshifter motif of enantiodromia, the process of turning into its opposite.

Since the dream stages a drama of which Eamonn is the producer, director, script writer and only actor, the aggression is really coming at him from the collective level in his own unconscious. He says very generally, 'people got aggressive with me', which suggests that it's a parental or societal injunction that violently doesn't approve of his gambling.

The dream draws this conflict – happiness versus aggression – to Eamonn's attention, asking him to do something about the problem. He feels he has to escape from the betting shop, otherwise he'd 'be injured'. That's the unconscious presentation, what has registered deep inside, so Eamonn has some conscious thinking to do about this situation. He needs to evaluate if gambling is as problematic for him as the dream suggests. Certainly by making a decision about whether it is a problem, and plumping for one side of the conflict or the other – to gamble or not to gamble –

will cause both the conflict and the subsequent 'state' Eamonn finds himself in to disappear. But will that one-sided approach work towards his salvation or destruction?

It's important to remember that our unconscious has our own best interests at heart, and that this dream has been presented to Eamonn for a reason. There's a definite warning in this dream from the Trickster or Shapeshifter motif. Part of the waking up for Eamonn is to consciously take the warning on board, accept being tricked into his better half, and finally do something practical about the problem.

Hugh's dream of doing the Leaving Cert

✦ ✧ ✦ ✧ ✦

I dreamt I was back doing the Leaving Cert in my old school. I was sitting at my old desk, which was too small for me, and I was my present age – 40, whereas everyone else was around 18. I hadn't prepared for it, and I couldn't remember how to answer the maths questions. I woke up in a panic. – Hugh

✦ ✧ ✦ ✧ ✦

The Leaving Cert is arguably the most stressful examination that any of us will ever have to face, because the results have the power to dictate our future path in an unprecedented way. And while we would have been able to attempt the maths questions at 18 years of age, if we were presented with the same questions 20 years later, it's conceivable that we will have forgotten how to do them. If, in addition, we hadn't prepared for the examination, then we're facing potential failure. And failure causes us to panic.

The bottom line in this dream is that Hugh, at 40 years of age, is undergoing a test that's more appropriate for an 18-year-old. He's sitting at his old desk in his old school, and the desk is now too small for him. Manifestly Hugh is too old to be in this situation, and he has grown beyond it. He hasn't prepared for it, he can't remember how to do it, and the feelings of panic in the dream cause him to wake up, mercifully bringing this nightmare scenario to an end.

The ages that Hugh quotes in his dream are revealing. The age of 18 is the time we leave school and go out into the world to take up a job or to go to college, while the age of 40 marks the midlife transition when we will have accomplished the extraverted tasks of finding a suitable career, meeting a soulmate, setting up house, starting a family. Midlife is the time we face the more introverted 'what's next' question, or consider 'what is it all about, really'.

These times of transition are important to negotiate successfully, because they lay the foundation for what's to come. The dream draws to Hugh's attention in a forceful manner that he's relying on skills that are more appropriate to an 18-year-old in order to manage this situation, and such tools no longer work for a 40-year-old. Hugh will have learned a great deal about life in the 20 years since he left school, and that's the present-day wisdom he's now meant to draw on, not, for example, being able to answer abstruse maths questions from the Leaving Cert, which belongs firmly to the past. (I wonder how often in those intervening 20 years has Hugh been asked about how he did in maths in the Leaving, which tells another truth!).

The dream also says that Hugh isn't prepared for this transition, and a degree of panic is perhaps appropriate to get him to wake up to this situation, and to put in some proper preparatory work immediately. There's a principle in life that says it's never too late: you can always do something on the pitch until the final whistle blows.

To conclude, what has triggered this dream? Is there a job interview in the offing, does Hugh have to make a presentation at work, or is the dream pointing to difficulties in his emotional life that have caused him to regress to being a teenager? Whatever it is, Hugh should face up to the difficulty, because his unconscious is already onto the case and will continue to support him with its resources as he prepares appropriately for what's to come, so he can move forward courageously with the midlife transition stage of his personal journey.

Kathleen's dream of a pale blue mermaid

❧ ✧ ❧ ✧ ❧

I have a recurring dream that I'm in the back of my aunt's jeep while she's driving. A pale blue mermaid is dragging me under the bottom of the car, and I don't have the strength to kick, and my body won't allow me to scream. – Kathleen

❧ ✧ ❧ ✧ ❧

A mermaid is a fabulous marine creature, half woman and half fish, closely aligned with the feared sirens from Greek mythology, who were said to render mariners helpless with their song. Kathleen's mermaid is a version of the nightmare, the evil female spirit who held sleepers down and afflicted them with a feeling of suffocation. Here, Kathleen says, 'A pale blue mermaid is dragging me under the bottom of the car': the mermaid is dragging her into the suffocating depths. She continues, 'I don't have the strength to kick, and my body won't allow me to scream.' So Kathleen is physically helpless, and she's unable to call for help, which is a nightmare scenario.

The whole drama in Kathleen's dream is forcibly bringing to her attention that she isn't in control. She begins by describing herself as a passenger in the back of her aunt's jeep while her aunt is driving: Kathleen is not in the driving seat, rather she's in the position of a powerless child who has no input into what happens to her. And she's being driven by a representative of her parents' generation, with their attendant outlook, strictures and admonitions.

So the question is, what has happened in Kathleen's life to render her so powerless and childlike? What is happening in her everyday life that she feels she doesn't have the strength to kick back, to give voice to say stop or even to call for help?

Kathleen says this is a recurring dream, so this Shadow situation to do with her femininity has been going on for a long time in her life. The mermaid, her aunt and Kathleen are all female, and represent the three stages of femininity: the mermaid is the maiden in fairy tales, Kathleen is in the child position, and her aunt is the crone, the old woman doing the driving. The dream suggests that Kathleen needs to move on from being the child taking the back seat, and, unlikely as it may seem, to face the transition of going with the maiden, a scenario that appears frightening because the mermaid has Shadow qualities since she's dragging Kathleen under.

Urgent change is needed before the nightmare quality of this dream will begin to dissipate. So Kathleen needs to take whatever steps she can – no matter how small – to get herself out of this powerless situation that the dream paints for her attention. She needs to take some forceful decisions, no matter how unladylike, to get back into the driving seat of her life. When she makes decisions, she defines herself and takes charge of her own path. Making decisions will move her away from the myriad possibilities in fantasy that never get realised, and never come to fruition. Before she knows it, she will be well down the road to recovery.

The colour symbolism in this dream puts a positive gloss on this fearful situation, because it gives us the feeling tone. Kathleen says that the mermaid is 'pale blue'. In symbolism, a pale blue colour equates to peace, prudence and a serene conscience. Maybe what Kathleen most fears – perhaps a creative encounter with the depths of her unconscious in which a mermaid can swim happily – paradoxically will result in the most fruitful outcome. Play is the most creative activity we can engage in, so she should paint her dream, write about it, make music that expresses it, and let her unconscious have its sway. Our unconscious and its productions work for our autonomy, where we can live under our own self-directed laws and become independent. So Kathleen should just use her prudence, which involves foresight and practical wisdom, and soon her serene conscience, particularly if it has been formed by her aunt's generation, will become more appropriately up to date!

Laura's dream of something holding her down

✦ ✧ ✦ ✧ ✦

I dream that something is holding me down, but I'm trying to fight them off, but I can't. It's a terrifying figure. I wake up really freaked out. – Laura

✦ ✧ ✦ ✧ ✦

*W*hat is the metaphor in this dream? Laura says, 'something is holding me down', which is a metaphor for something that's occurring in her everyday life.

The dream presents as a typical nightmare, where there's a sensation while we sleep of a female figure sitting heavily on our chest. It also draws on the case of a mythological evil demon called an incubus, which lies on women and is reputed to have sex with them. Laura says, 'I'm trying to fight them off, but I can't'. And 'them' or the 'figure' terrifies her, so that she wakes up 'really freaked out'. The Shadow in women's dreams can often appear as a collective. The origins of the word 'freak' refer to a remarkable creature or being, which is both an angel and a demon, who has overtones of capriciousness or whimsy, and which earlier in the word's etymology referred to horror, shivering or the raising of hackles.

The first question is: what is holding Laura down? The dream presents this drama to her in nightmare form because her unconscious regards what's happening to her as being very serious, and it's screaming at her to pay attention. Another question is: what is it in Laura's daily life makes her feel so powerless? And finally: why does this predicament terrify her so?

On the collective level, Laura says that she is 'trying to fight them off', and then she says, 'It's a terrifying figure.' In the language of dreams and the unconscious, there's no binary contradiction here between plural and singular. She is saying that this Shadow figure is on the collective level of her parents or of society, which she finds terrifying to encounter.

If Laura can answer any or all of these questions, she will have gone some way towards finding a solution to the predicament in which she find herself. And she will be robbing the dream of the power it has over her so she will no longer awaken 'freaked out' because she will no longer be having these nightmares.

By confronting what Laura most fears, she will have taken a major step towards strengthening her angelic side in her personality, as well as the demonic. Both belong to her, and both should be allowed to have their say, as much as she can bear! By bringing such balance into her life, this nightmare will lose its power, she will have restful sleep at night, and she will experience an influx of energy during her waking hours.

Jarlath's dream of being thrown around the room

✦ ✧ ✦ ✧ ✦

I have a dream that I'm being thrown around the room by an invisible force while sleeping, and can't move. – Jarlath

✦ ✧ ✦ ✧ ✦

While we're sleeping, there's a mechanism at work in our bodies that inhibits us from getting up out of bed and acting out our dreams. And to a certain extent, that's what's happening in Jarlath's dream: as he says, 'I'm being thrown around the room by an invisible force while sleeping and can't move.' So at some level, while sleeping, Jarlath is aware of this mechanism that forbids movement. The ultimate aim is to preserve sleep, and to keep Jarlath asleep.

There's also an echo here of a much earlier time in Jarlath's life – a body memory, if you like. When we were babies and young children, we were moved about by our mothers or fathers whether we liked it or not. And of course as infants we couldn't move.

Finally, there's also a nightmarish quality about Jarlath's dream: 'I'm being thrown around the room by an invisible force … and can't move.' This tells us that Jarlath feels helpless, overpowered by something.

A dream is a metaphor for something, and it tries to bring this to our attention. So I'd ask Jarlath, 'What is it in your life that has you in its power, rather than you as an adult being in control of it? What is this force that's normally hidden from others or from yourself?' The word 'force' is grounded in strength. So there's a strong, hidden power in action in Jarlath's life that is throwing him.

Jarlath says he 'can't move'. What is that situation drawing to his attention? That he's afraid to move, or that he feels he is in a checkmate position? Whatever it is, Jarlath needs to take the necessary preparatory steps that will enable him to make a move eventually in his own way and at his own pace.

The dream is an unconscious presentation, but Jarlath has to bring his consciousness to bear on the dream as well. Out of the combination of the unconscious and the conscious, he can arrive at a new third position, which is neither one nor the other, but partakes of both. That's the more balanced position which has yet to be achieved, and towards which the nightmare drama of this dream is pointing.

Kieran's dream of being in a nightclub

♦ ✧ ♦ ✧ ♦

I was in a nightclub. Everyone was really drunk and I couldn't find my friends. I had lost my wallet and had to get out, but was trapped. Next thing I'm chased by a pack of wolves. I woke up in a sweat. – Kieran

♦ ✧ ♦ ✧ ♦

This is a nightmare, which means that the dream is shouting at Kieran to pay attention. The drama of the dream paints a picture of Kieran being trapped. The word 'trapped' originally was applied to an animal caught in a snare or a pitfall, and Kieran says he 'had to get out, but was trapped'. His whole psyche is reacting to the truth of the situation: it doesn't like the club scene. As Kieran describes it, 'everyone was really drunk'; not a little merry, but really drunk, and 'everyone' presumably includes Kieran himself. He couldn't find his friends, so he was on his own, without support. He'd lost his wallet, so he had no means of looking after himself or paying for help. Kieran was abandoned and isolated, and he concluded that he 'had to get out'.

Whether it's the clubbing scene or the drink that is the problem, Kieran is being asked to pay attention to the situation he finds himself in, and to do something about it. According to the dream, he has to get out. Kieran says he 'woke up in a sweat', but at least he has woken up to this situation, and hopefully he will take steps to inaugurate change before matters deteriorate even further.

The final act in the dream after Kieran is trapped is that he says, 'I'm chased by a pack of wolves'. Wolves are predators and are an ancient source of fear for mankind. They occur in myths, legends and fairy tales, for example, in the tale of Little Red Riding Hood and the Wolf. So in the final act, the dream underlines for Kieran, on the deepest mythological level, that unless he takes this dream seriously, he will be devoured – maybe by the addiction of drink, which seems to underlie what's happening in the nightclub.

A pack of wolves is a collective, normally a supportive family group led by an alpha male and female. On another level, perhaps Kieran is being chased by prohibitions imposed by his parents, family or society, or even by his own conscience, which was formed in conjunction with all of these.

So Kieran needs to stay awake to the predicament he is in and, if necessary, cut out the drink, go to Alcoholics Anonymous and get the support that he needs. Then he'll have a healthy and happy life of freedom, as opposed to one where he feels trapped, with no way out. In any case, he needs to honour his dream!

Nora's dream of being possessed

✦ ✧ ✦ ✧ ✦

I had a dream that I was possessed. I could feel whatever it was inside my body and I had to perform the exorcism myself. I was half awake and could feel every bit of it, even though I literally could not move my body. I've had this dream four times. – Nora

✦ ✧ ✦ ✧ ✦

This is a nightmare of immobility that's fairly common, and Nora says she's had it four times. The dreamer dreams they're half-awake but they can't move their body; they're petrified, turned to stone. It's part of the sleeping process where we lose our ability to move. While Nora becomes aware of this process in her dream, her sleeping is still preserved: she doesn't get up and sleepwalk, for example. So Nora's body is functioning properly. Essentially Nora is trying to wake herself up, to be consciously in charge of herself once again, but her body is putting up a real fight to stay asleep and to be immobile. And the dream expresses the battle taking place between two opposing instincts: the death instinct expressed by the desire to keep sleeping, and the life instinct that wants to wake up.

The opening line of Nora's dream is 'I had a dream that I was possessed.' Drawing on medieval religious imagery, she expands on this idea and says, 'I could feel whatever it was inside my body, and I had to perform the exorcism myself.' In other words, she had to drive out an evil spirit by prayers and ceremonies. Nora felt that there was something alien inside her that she experienced as evil, and that she needed to perform a ritual action in order to come back to herself. The question is: what is Nora experiencing that she feels is so bad, wicked or vicious as to evoke the drama of this dream?

Interestingly, possession comes from the Latin word '*potis*', meaning being able, or having mastery. This drama is a metaphor for the fact that Nora wants to be a fully functioning subject, rather than be subjected to the will of another. But this battle is primarily taking place inside her, and she should examine the emotions and the feelings she repudiates so much that she experiences them as alien and as coming from outside to possess her. What positive aspects of them could she consciously incorporate in order to function in a less split-off manner? Badness or wickedness have elements of self-affirmation that are necessary and important for us, and viciousness has great, defensive strength. By making friends with our less edifying qualities, by incorporating our Shadow, we can become more truly ourselves. Nora says she had this dream four times. The number four signifies the wholeness or completeness towards which this dream is tending. It can only come about in our personalities when we embrace every aspect of ourselves, which means finding a home for our Shadow side, as well as for our goodness.

Lorcan's dream of a post-apocalyptic Ireland

✦ ✧ ✦ ✧ ✦

I had a dream that I was in a post-apocalyptic Ireland. Everyone was in rags and there was no food or water. I felt alone and scared. There were crazed zombies eating people alive. – Lorcan

✦ ✧ ✦ ✧ ✦

What do we feel from reading about the horrific reality of Lorcan's dream? A good aid when trying to understand a dream and heighten its effect is to insert the words 'and this is my life' at the end of every sentence. Lorcan says, 'I was in a post-apocalyptic Ireland [and this is my life]. Everyone was in rags, and there was no food or water [and this is my life].' Yes, something so disastrous has happened where Lorcan lives that it has destroyed everything, and there's nothing left to support life.

The psychotic effects of such a trauma are visible in the dream: 'There were crazed zombies eating people alive [and this is my life].' In the voodoo cult, a zombie is a corpse brought back to life. And these zombies in Lorcan's dream were also crazed, or driven mad, insane. Rightly, Lorcan says he 'felt alone and scared', which is the important sentence in this dream, because his unconscious is reacting to a current situation in which he finds himself. At some profound level, Lorcan's world has been destroyed, and where he is now is an alien situation for him. He feels all by himself, and under existential threat.

The dream brings this situation to Lorcan's attention in nightmare form because his unconscious regards it as being of the utmost urgency; it's a problem that needs to be tackled immediately. Lorcan needs to reach out to someone he can trust and tell them what's going on for him, so that he can feel supported and not be so alone and scared. Sometimes our problems are so overwhelming that we can't see a way out. Problems can have an obvious solution for someone who isn't so caught up in them and who has an expertise that we may not have. So Lorcan needs to ask for help in dealing with his devastating situation. He should talk to someone he can trust, like his family doctor.

The dream he describes should be brought to a reputable therapist, if that's possible for him, because it has features that are worrying, for example, 'a post-apocalyptic Ireland'. 'Apocalypse' is a Middle English word meaning a vision or hallucination, from a Latin and Greek word meaning revelation: literally, an uncovering. So it refers to a vision or prophecy, especially of violent or climactic events. An apocalypse is a revelation of a future upheaval where something is uncovered, in a dream for example. Lorcan's dream isn't a prediction, but it has warning elements in it, such as 'crazed zombies eating people alive'. In order to avoid being devoured by that zombie part of himself, Lorcan needs to break out of that 'alone' feeling and ask for help with whatever is so grievously distressing him.

Finally, it's important to emphasise that the dream is showing that a part of him has survived this apocalypse. While this survival may not be sustainable in the longer term – 'there was no food or water' – at the moment he has survived and come through, and that should be a source of great consolation. But Lorcan does need outside intervention to support him in coming to terms with what has happened to him, and to help him find a direction that will work for him in going forward with his life.

Orlaith's dream of the end of the world

✦ ✧ ✦ ✧ ✦

In my dream, I was driving up a narrow back road. On both sides of the road there were burned out cars upside down. It felt like the end of the world. – Orlaith

✦ ✧ ✦ ✧ ✦

What a calamitous feeling to have arising out of a dream: 'It felt like the end of the world', the end of everything. For human beings, our consciousness equates the end of the world with death. Orlaith has had intimations of mortality visiting her in her dream. I wonder what gave rise to that? Normally, some elements in a dream would be a reworking of material from the day before. Could this have arisen from images that Orlaith might have seen on television, or is the dream a representation of something from her past?

The drama of Orlaith's dream is interesting. She's in the driving seat. So Orlaith is in control, which is a positive element in this dream. She says that on both sides of the road there were burned out cars upside down. There was a lot of destruction and detritus you'd see in the aftermath of a war, for example, showing terrible damage. In nature fire is transformative, destroying foliage to make way for new life. But here the fire from man-made machines was destructive, which adds to the feeling of disaster.

If we were to take the phrase that Orlaith uses – 'it felt like the end of the world' – and place it back along the timeline of her life, where would that feeling of disaster apply? Where in her life was there terrible damage that resulted in a lot of destruction? It's important to emphasise that Orlaith has survived that. In the dream she's a survivor looking at the aftermath; there's no sense that her car is going to be burned out and turned upside down.

In dreams a car can indicate the way we move through the various activities of life. So here it appears as if at some time in the past, something Orlaith experienced turned things upside down and stopped progress. The horsepower of her life, the energy she uses to get herself from a to b, was so seriously compromised that she felt as if her world had come to an end. For some reason, her unconscious dream-life is reminding her of that destructive time, maybe to help her in realising that she's a survivor, that she has triumphed, and that her present need not be coloured so entirely by her past. As the dream says, Orlaith is driving up a narrow back road and not on the main highway, so it is important now to place her experience in that minor context so she can move onwards and upwards!

Patricia's dream of a public beheading

✦ ✧ ✦ ✧ ✦

I had a dream that I was in a medieval England type of place. The streets were filthy and there were horses racing along the streets. Then there was a public beheading, with cheering crowds. The head was held up and it was my sister! I woke up screaming. – Patricia

✦ ✧ ✦ ✧ ✦

What a shocking nightmare to have. Patricia says she woke up screaming at the recognition of the terrible fate that befell her sister. Patricia has witnessed something primitive and medieval – streets filthy, horses racing in the streets, a public beheading with cheering crowds.

The use of the word 'horse' usually denotes something inferior, coarse or unrefined. Horsepower is a common unit of power measurement, so there's a great deal of energy contained in these horses racing in filthy streets in this dream, which has also the inferior feeling of the Trickster about it. I wonder if this could be a reaction to the horror of recent terrorist attacks caused by Isil, and their barbaric treatment of people they consider different to themselves – the beheadings we've heard about on television and radio. The medieval barbarism of a public beheading in Patricia's dream relates to her sister, which Patricia experiences as being so unbearable that she wakes up screaming.

We have no experience of our own death; we only experience death through the deaths of others. It could be that Patricia's empathy towards her sister (as they share the same gene pool) is a realisation that the medieval barbarism she experiences in the dream could also be practised towards herself; that she, too, is at risk of an arbitrary and summary form of injustice, and we don't know the day nor the hour when death will come to us. So the dream posits for Patricia in a graphic manner the horror and finality of death.

We should also ask is there anyone in Patricia's immediate surroundings who would arbitrarily assault her, who bears ill will towards her, or who would kill her if they could? 'I'll kill her' is a metaphorical phrase that we may have heard from our parents, and perhaps that we also use in relation to others at a less mature, middle age in our lives before enlightenment, which is a further application of Patricia's use of the word medieval: Latin *medium aevum*.

Finally, it would be worth Patricia examining the aggressive feelings she has towards her sister, perhaps feelings of sibling rivalry, where she could 'cut the head off her', to use a common phrase. Every part of our dream gives our personalities a voice, and our feelings towards others are always ambivalent: we both love and hate people. As Patricia describes in her dream, she was in 'a medieval England type of place', which underlines the more primitive and less developed part of her personality.

Patricia's description, 'I woke up screaming [when the head was held up]', suggests that when the dream confronted her with her unconscious reality, she both recognised and was horrified by what she saw. Our Shadow isn't pleasant! If Patricia were to make these hidden, primitive and unconscious wishes more conscious, then there's less likelihood of her acting them out and scapegoating her sister.

Patricia must let the dream deepen her understanding of the human nature we all share, and be grateful that she lives in a liberal democracy. It's worth defending against those who operate out of any form of rigid fundamentalism, which cannot accommodate difference or tolerate ambivalence, especially their own.

Róisín's dream of having murdered someone

✦ ❖ ✦ ❖ ✦

In my dream I have murdered someone. In every dream that has happened since, the police are getting closer to finding out I'm the killer. – Róisín

✦ ❖ ✦ ❖ ✦

Róisín is being persecuted by guilt. She says, 'in every dream that has happened since', meaning that this nightmare of anxiety repeats in her unconscious. It continually presents this scenario to her in dream form so that she can deal with the problem. Róisín says 'the police are getting closer to finding out', so this repetition is, in fact, a dream series, moving inexorably towards the conclusion that Róisín will be exposed as 'the killer'.

Every problem in life can be solved or dealt with in some way, with the exception of death. So to take another person's life, to deprive another human being of their life, ultimately all that they have, is regarded as the greatest crime there is. In her dream Róisín accuses herself of having committed this unforgivable act, of being the killer. So at a very deep level of her unconscious, Róisín believes she has done this, and she can't forgive herself.

She also says, 'the police are getting closer to finding out I'm the killer', which implies that she hasn't owned up to the crime and is keeping it a secret. Róisín begins her dream with the sentence 'I have murdered someone'. Today the word 'murder' refers to a criminal homicide, but it's a very old word, and originally it meant the secret killing of a person. Róisín's dream expresses the truth that – on top of the actual act of murder – the burden of the secret sets her apart from her participation in human affairs, because secrets are poisonously isolating.

Guilt comes from an internal conflict at having done something we shouldn't have done. Essentially it comes from not having lived up to parental expectations, and it has its beginnings at a time when we were very small, when we internalised our parents' reactions. The result is that we think if we feel guilty, then we must be guilty!

Figuratively, murder refers to great wickedness. So very early on in her life, Róisín must have done something that she considered so wicked and evil that she feels it was as bad as committing murder. She believes she is a killer, and the parental police are getting close to finding out her secret: that she's a murderer.

It will help if Róisín can examine her conscience, and see if she can remember what the worst thing was she ever did as a child. This memory may be hedged around with taboos, and Róisín may have some difficulty going back there. But just as we were terrified of what lurked in the wardrobe or in the cupboard under the stairs in the dark, when we go back and look at these shadow areas from an adult's perspective, we realise there's nothing there and that we were haunted simply by the phantoms of our imagination. Róisín, too, will be able to see that her behaviour at the time was just a child being a child who happened to collide with a parent's frustration, hangover or even cruelty. Hopefully, Róisín will be able to laugh at what she discovers and believed was a wrongful act, be able to forgive herself and suffer no more nightmares to do with guilt.

Finally, it would also help if Róisín were to draw a list of those she would like to metaphorically 'murder'! We don't like to acknowledge our aggression and anger, and yet these emotions have an important, protective function in our lives. Since we cannot be rid of them, we try to hide them from ourselves and from others. So Róisín should let those feelings surface and examine where the seam of anger and aggression runs in her life today, even if its manifestation is just a slight, irritable perturbation. If she acknowledges and owns her murderous feelings and the guilt she feels in relation to them, she will be able to embrace her killer instinct and use it appropriately whenever and wherever necessary!

Sheila's dream of a figure standing over her in bed

✦ ✧ ✦ ✧ ✦

I dream that I'm woken by a figure standing over me in bed. I can't see their face. I feel a rush of fear and panic. I wake up just as the figure's hands start closing around me to take me away. It looks like the grim reaper. Is this a bad omen? – Sheila

✦ ✧ ✦ ✧ ✦

An omen is a sign of what's going to happen, a prediction, and while a dream can do that – most notably the account of Abraham Lincoln's dream of a president's funeral in the White House a fortnight before he was assassinated – normally an unconscious presentation in the form of a dream should always be engaged with consciously. That way we can arrive at a third position that partakes of both the unconscious and consciousness. In Sheila's dream, she says, 'I wake up', so hopefully she will pay attention to what the dream is trying to say to her in pictorial language.

Sheila says, 'I dream that I'm woken by a figure standing over me'. To stand over a person is an intimidating gesture of power, designed to watch or exercise control over them. This happens for Sheila in her bedroom, normally a private place of vulnerability and intimacy. Her reaction to this extraordinary situation is a rush of fear and panic, which is an appropriate reaction to that space being invaded by a figure – a shape or a form. She continues: 'I can't see their face.' In the western world, we read people's faces, and we don't like them to be obscured because we find it threatening. In Sheila's dream, this threat is increased exponentially by the hands closing in around her to take her away, and further increased by her association of the figure to the grim reaper, or the personification of death. So the energy in Sheila's dream is coming ultimately from a fear of death. 'Is this a bad omen?' she asks. Well, we are all going to die one day, but hopefully for most of us, not in the immediate future!

Something unwanted and unwarranted must have happened to Sheila in the previous 24 hours to trigger such an invasive dream, in which Sheila feels so intruded upon that she feels threatened and helpless. The dream draws on images from her childhood of someone standing over her, closing in around her to take her away, without her having given them permission. The paradigm for this type of dream comes from our parents. When we were little, they stood over us when we were sleeping, and sometimes their hands might close in around us to take us away, to move us from the car to bed, or from one room to another. So have her parents, her boss at work or even her partner approached her in such an uninvited and unwanted way that Sheila's unconscious is reacting violently to this undermining occurrence?

The dream paints a picture for Sheila of her unconscious helplessness in nightmare form in order to urge her consciousness not to allow her to be railroaded as if she were a child, and to fight back for her autonomy. If Sheila succeeds in this endeavour, then the dream won't turn out to be a bad omen.

Michael's dream about a woman hanging outside the window

✦ ✧ ✦ ✧ ✦

I dreamt that I woke up and tried to scream but no noise came out. I tried to turn on the side lamp but the bulb had been unscrewed slightly. I opened the blind, and there was a woman hanging outside the window. She was hanging like a woman on the front of a ship on a mast kind of thing. I then woke up. What on earth? – Michael

✦ ✧ ✦ ✧ ✦

There's a nightmare quality to this dream: as Michael says, 'I woke up and tried to scream, but no noise came out'. Michael is so terrified by something that he tries to scream, but finds he's unable. 'I tried to turn on the side lamp, but the bulb had been unscrewed slightly' – so he can't throw light on this situation either. In these opening two sentences, Michael tests his ability to perform, and he suffers failure on both occasions.

It's also important to state that the word 'nightmare' originally meant an evil female spirit who supposedly had sexual intercourse with the sleeper. There's also a sexual component in every dream. Purely from that perspective, Michael uses the word 'screwed', which is coarse slang for sexual intercourse. It appears in the dream when Michael talks about the bulb having been unscrewed slightly. The bulb is an object with a rounded, swollen top like the glans of a penis. It failed because it had been unscrewed from the hole. And the original meaning of the word 'screw' referred to the cylinder or hole in which the screw turned – so figuratively, the vagina.

When Michael opens the blind, there's a woman hanging outside the window. He then corrects himself and says, 'hanging like a woman on the front of a ship on a mast kind of thing'. Figureheads draped over the prow of a ship were often naked women with their breasts exposed, but what Michael actually said was that she was 'hanging like a woman … on a mast kind of thing'. A mast is a long upright pole on a ship to support the sails and rigging. However, Michael is most probably referring to the bowsprit here, which is a stout pole or beam extending out from the prow – penis-like! So the image is of a woman impaled by a long extended pole being 'screwed'.

After all of this, Michael says, 'I then woke up,' and he asks, 'What on earth?' This is an emphatic question: Michael woke up to what? It's possible that the drama of the dream could be staging a scene of Michael watching porn on his laptop: 'I opened the blind, and there was a woman hanging outside the window.' He's separated from this woman by the glass of the window, so there's no personal connection between them, and it also implies that he's unable to have full intercourse. So he says, 'I tried to turn on the side lamp … but the bulb had been unscrewed slightly'. The adjective 'slightly' means slender, flimsy, small and unimportant. Again, Michael's effort at sex 'on the side' was unsuccessful.

What's traumatising and terrifying for Michael, as described in his dream, is the failure of his sexual prowess. It has echoes of an earlier time, in the formation of his Oedipus complex, which was mythologised by Freud as the time that the child realises for the first time that his puny penis can never satisfy his first love object, his mother; that he's in fact inadequate in the penis department. In this opening salvo of the battle of the sexes, the child's father always wins. The realisation for the child of this fault line is a huge and terrifying let-down. The acceptance of this lack, limitation and loss is a paradigm for all of us to successfully weather the many experiences of failure that we will face in our lives. If Michael can reconcile with these three 'l's – lack, limitation and loss – the dream will have accomplished its work, and he will be the more psychologically mature because of it.

Tina's dream about a woman falling down a lift shaft

◆ ◇ ◆ ◇ ◆

Last night I dreamt that I stepped into a lift, and a woman was in there. The lift was rocky and it fell apart, with the woman falling down the shaft. Someone then shot her. I woke up! — a freaked out Tina

◆ ◇ ◆ ◇ ◆

This is a nightmare in which Tina wakes up and is 'freaked out'. The slang phrase 'freaked out' only came into use 50 years ago, and it means to become excited or stimulated by drugs. It comes from the noun 'freak', which refers to an habitual user of drugs. From this perspective, a lift from drugs can take you high, and it can also take you down into the depths of the fear. Is that at play, I wonder?

What do we make of the drama of the dream, and in particular the fact that Tina steps into the lift, and that's the last we hear of her? Since this is Tina's dream, it's all about her: she wrote the script, she cast the characters and she constructed the drama, so every aspect of this dream refers to Tina. In her dream, she has cast herself in the role of observer – moving from the first to the third person – to protect herself from the horrifying aspects of the ensuing drama. However, like the woman already in there, she has 'stepped into the lift' too.

The essence of the drama seems to be that something that is designed to support us and take us to where we want to go – a lift – fails spectacularly. The emotive words Tina employs to describe what happened to her support are 'rocky' and 'it fell apart'. And her reaction to this unhappy situation is 'falling down' and 'shot'. The verb 'to fall' is important here as the use of 'fell apart' and 'falling down' register in the unconscious as equivalents, and are describing a person's downfall. The woman in the lift is clearly an aspect of Tina who is no longer supported: she's rocky, falling apart and falling down. If that weren't bad enough, she is shot at the conclusion of this drama. So in her dream Tina paints a picture where an aspect of herself – the 'woman' – is let down very badly and is under attack.

A shaft is a vertical space – figuratively, a vagina – and also a long slender rod or pole, slang for a penis. The word 'shot' means the discharge of a gun. So in her dream, Tina describes an act of sexual intercourse, which has her freaked out.

Where in her life does Tina not feel supported as a woman? Where does she feel under attack, sexually and otherwise? She doesn't tell us. But at least she's waking up to this situation, although it's freaking her out since it's coming to her in nightmare form, because the unconscious wants her to pay attention to what's happening and to mobilise her psychic energy to do something about it. In other words, the dream is asking Tina to put more solid supports in place so that she won't feel so literally let down and unsupported.

Niall's dream about being at a gig

✦ ✧ ✦ ✧ ✦

I dreamt that I was at a gig and everyone was on their mobile phones. It was like they were all zombies. My girlfriend was shouting gibberish at me. Everything was loud and scary, and I woke in a sweat. – Niall

✦ ✧ ✦ ✧ ✦

This is a dream about the alienation that we all can experience. The drama of Niall's dream is showing a disconnect between Niall and the others in his circle. His unconscious employs the modern phenomenon of everyone being on their mobile phones to illustrate this point, and presumably they were not speaking, just texting. He says, 'It was like they were all zombies.' A zombie is a corpse brought back to life, and the transferred sense is to be stupefied or lethargic. The result was that nobody was available to relate to him. Even his girlfriend was shouting senseless chatter 'at me'. This tells us there was no conversation because Niall's girlfriend didn't seek any response from him.

Niall says, 'Everything was loud and scary'. It was scary because there was no possibility of human contact; nobody was making a connection with him. Of vital importance here is the unstated picture that emerges from the dream: neither was it possible for Niall to communicate. Nobody could hear him because of the loudness. So the dream paints a graphic picture of Niall's isolation, which is a dangerous position to be in. If he cannot be heard, he could act out in order to draw somebody's attention in a violent manner to what he has to say. And that is the meaning in this nightmare.

The question is: what has triggered this alienation and isolation to the extent that Niall can't even understand his girlfriend? And why is Niall's unconscious bringing this breakdown in communication to his attention now? Obviously Niall needs to do something about this, and maybe there's a clue in the opening line of his dream: 'I dreamt that I was at a gig'. Dare I suggest that such a venue is not the ideal location to connect up with people in a meaningful way. People are focused on the music and the musicians, they could be out of it on drugs or drink, it's too loud to favour speech, and for many other reasons, the environment of a gig doesn't favour meaningful conversation.

Niall is asked to make a soft and unthreatening space available in his world for communication, and to calm down his life so that he has the time to make meaningful connections with people, in his own way and at his own pace. Since everyone in a dream expresses an aspect of the dreamer's personality, Niall himself is included in this collective act of everyone being on their mobile phones. There's a warning here about technology that Niall needs to take to heart. He should give consideration to a technological sunset, and switch everything off from time to time. This will give him the opportunity to find out that an unmediated give and take with others will be so infinitely rewarding that he will no longer wake 'in a sweat' or have nightmares about not being able to speak.

Una's dream of being trapped with an evil old lady

✦ ✧ ✦ ✧ ✦

I dreamt of being trapped on a staircase with an evil old lady about to attack me! What does this mean? – Una

✦ ✧ ✦ ✧ ✦

Una describes an old lady about to attack her. What do we hear in that description? Yes, Una is talking about her mother, or at least a woman who holds the symbolic position of her mother in her consciousness – it could even be a female boss who has old or outdated attitudes. And she further qualifies this by calling the old lady 'evil', which is a very early English word dating from about 700, meaning bad, wicked or vicious. So it's quite clear that Una is allergic to this person. As she says, 'I dreamt of being trapped on a staircase with an evil old lady about to attack me.' Una isn't actually attacked by the old lady; she's about to be attacked, and her unconscious is bringing this to her attention because the attack is something she fears will happen in the future.

There are two questions arising out of this dream. Where in her life does Una feel trapped by her mother, or a substitute for her mother? And why does she feel that her mother would be about to attack her; what sin has she committed that has caused her mother's wrath to be about to descend on her?

The geography of this dream is interesting. Una says that she is 'trapped on a staircase'. A staircase leads both up and down. There are actually two exits; two choices that Una can make to get away. She is not trapped in a room with only one door or an exit that is blocked.

So Una needs to chose an exit, free herself from her mother and move on with her life. Life is far too short to put up with being trapped, especially by an older version of herself – her mother – that she experiences as being bad, wicked and vicious! While her mother has a hook on which she can hang the quality 'evil', Una should examine whether aspects of that description could possibly be applied to herself as well, even though she may not wish to acknowledge them. In working through that recognition, there's salvation and freedom. Una needs to live her own life in the here and now, embrace the freedom to be herself, and value the freedom from traditional ways of doing things that such a commitment will bring.

9

Persona Dreams

*T*he word 'persona', taken from the Latin, refers to the masks that actors have worn in solemn ritual ceremonies and in drama across the world for thousands of years. We're all familiar with the comic and tragic masks of classical Greek drama, which we see today decorating the proscenium arch in theatres. Persona dreams make reference to the roles we play in everyday life, roles that smooth the way for us to survive when we're adapting to the demands of society.

There are two aspects to the Persona. On the one hand, we have our own personal identity and individual values, and on the other hand, there are social expectations that others – or life in general – can have of us. Our Persona enables us to adapt, so that we can find the best fit where both of these aspects, the personal and the public, can have a voice.

We need to have a flexible Persona so that we can be different people in different situations, at home and at work, for example. A mother's or father's Persona holds out to us certain principles or requirements that we know in advance. For example, the attitude that children come first, or that you just get on with things and do what has to be done. These convenient Persona signposts make our paths through life easier.

Parental expectations usually draw out our first Persona patterns, and that loving one-on-one interaction helps us to build a secure and individual Persona. Going to crèche or playschool then forces us to be social and to adapt to the collective.

If we haven't developed an adequate Persona, we will feel inept and vulnerable in public situations; we won't feel adequately protected from the rough and tumble of interacting with others. The expectations with which we're faced from the collective will seem overwhelming to us, and we'll be tempted to drop out.

The opposite Persona problem is where we identify with our role to such an extent that we're permanently on stage in character, be it as mother, surgeon, priest or president, without any personal values. A person can be an admirable and powerful public figure, but if he fails to be a human being, he is just a trapped stereotype limited by the parameters of his role, and destructively split off from the unutilised potential that makes him a unique individual.

Persona problems are often shown through the clothes we wear – or don't wear. When we maintain a Persona to the detriment of ourselves, we can often feel like a fraud or that we'll be found out. These problems show up in Persona dreams, which counsel us to bring more balance into the conflict we experience between our public and private selves.

Maura's dream of walking in public

✦ ✧ ✦ ✧ ✦

In my dream I'm walking in public, and suddenly my legs are heavy and stuck to the ground. I can't keep walking. I feel the pain of trying to pull and push my legs forward to move, but I can't. I wake up with sore legs and out of breath. Help please! – Maura

✦ ✧ ✦ ✧ ✦

Maura's dream is a fairly common nightmare in which we're stuck to the ground and can't move forward. This dream demonstrates the battle we all have to preserve sleep, which is one of the functions of dreams. On the one hand, we want to be asleep and immobile, and on the other, we have a desire to wake up and be fully conscious. This conflict is played out in Maura's dream to such an extent that, as she says, 'I wake up with sore legs and out of breath.'

Maura says, 'I'm walking in public', which means she is open to general observation, sight or knowledge, with the potential to be judged. The dream paints a picture for Maura of her walking in full view of everyone else, and suddenly she can't continue on – as Maura says, she's 'stuck to the ground'. So the dream brings a particular Persona problem to Maura's attention as well, which is coming at her in nightmare form in order that she can address it. When she's performing in public, Maura's Persona – the mask we put on when we go out to work, our professional face, if you like – isn't working for her as it should be, and the effect of this is that she grinds to a halt. Maura isn't able to continue walking, which is one of the first basic motor skills we learn as a child. In other words, Maura can't do the basics, and she's stuck to the ground out of fear, out of shyness, or more likely, out of self-consciousness.

The drama of the dream portrays Maura as having a social phobia, which is a fairly common form of anxiety disorder. The person experiences intense anxiety, as she puts it, 'in public', where he or she can be exposed to unfamiliar people or be subject to possible scrutiny or judgement.

Maura is obviously distressed by her dream and she appeals – 'Help please!' While her dream is trying to protect her sleep, it also draws to her attention that she suffers from social anxiety. So what are the societal judgements that are causing her pain as she tries to move forward in her life? What attitudes does she attribute to others that are holding her back? These judgements primarily come from herself; that's what the dream is showing her. It may be that the others, whoever they are, have a hook on which she has hung a particular interpretation of the law, since the word 'judgement' is a compound of *jus*, meaning 'right' or 'law', and the root *dicere*, meaning 'to say'. The general meaning is 'one who decides a question'. This judgement or interpretation has, in fact, come from Maura, since she can never be sure someone else shares her opinion without asking them. So Maura should examine herself and her opinions, and take back the judgements that she doesn't recognise as belonging to her. If she succeeds in this, she will not only help herself, but she will have made a major contribution to society as well. It's a truism that the greatest act we can do for humanity is to become healthy and mature human beings ourselves, and withdrawing our projections onto others is a necessary part of that process.

All of our phobias should be challenged to the utmost extent that we can bear. They can be challenged in our own way, and at our own pace, so that we feel we're in control. If Maura takes measures to address and confront this problem – if she becomes less self-conscious in public – she will stop having this type of nightmare, and more importantly, she will be able to move forward in her life with ease. Our Persona is there to ease our various social interactions, but it's not meant to be a burden that weighs us down; it can be worn lightly, which ultimately is our choice.

Iseult's dream of ending up in public in her underwear

✦ ✧ ✦ ✧ ✦

I have this dream that I end up in public in my underwear. I've been having it for years. I wake up feeling panicked and embarrassed. – Iseult

✦ ✧ ✦ ✧ ✦

*I*seult says that in her dream 'I end up in public in my underwear'. It's clear from this dream that her public Persona isn't working. Despite her best efforts, she ends up not properly dressed outside, where she feels exposed and vulnerable: she needs more protection. There's also a strong suggestion that despite her best efforts, the end result is that she's virtually naked in public. While it may be alright to go around the house – our private space – in our underwear, when we go out into the street there's a social expectation that we should be properly dressed. Iseult continues: 'I wake up feeling panicked and embarrassed.' So she's very uncomfortable with the situation in which she finds herself.

Iseult says, 'I've been having this dream for years'. So this particular dream has been asking Iseult again and again to pay attention to her Persona problem, because she doesn't have an appropriate way of relating to others when she goes outside her home.

Iseult has to up her levels of security. Maybe she has to be more discreet, not share personal problems at work, nor let her personal life intrude into her work life. She needs to thoroughly examine where she feels vulnerable and open to attack in her daily life, and then go and tackle the problem so that she no longer feels panicked and embarrassed when she's in public. Although she may start out properly dressed, something happens when she's out there to expose her in public. What is that? What triggers that exposure?

Iseult uses a revealing verb: to 'end up'. The Indo-European root of that is the word 'boundary'. This strongly suggests that Iseult should put certain boundaries in place to protect her from feeling naked under the public scrutiny of others. We all need to retain a core of privacy, so in light of her dream, Iseult should be careful of how and with whom she shares her innermost self. Certainly she needs to be even more protective of her privacy than others would normally be, in order to definitively bring to an end what's happening to her in her dream.

Aileen's dream of going to work on roller skates

✦ ✧ ✦ ✧ ✦

I had a dream that I went to work on roller skates. I went around the office on them all day and no one batted an eye. Then my colleagues became cement and every time they touched, they got stuck together. – Aileen

✦ ✧ ✦ ✧ ✦

*A*ren't dreams just marvellous? It's amazing the way the unconscious paints pictures so that we can read the messages it's trying to get through to us! Since, for the most part, dreams are non-verbal, the unconscious communicates through dramatic images.

Aileen says that she 'went to work on roller skates'. That's right, she got her skates on at work; she made haste – and she says no one batted an eye. So she has permission to wear this Persona at work.

However, in the second half of her dream, her colleagues 'became cement', meaning they hardened into a rock-like substance. So as a result of Aileen getting her skates on, her colleagues slowed up so much that they actually turned to stone; they were petrified.

Finally, Aileen says that every time they touched, they 'got stuck together'. So I think the dream is telling Aileen that her colleagues will literally stick together if she makes haste at work; they will band together in being slow, in contradistinction to her. So given this warning in her dream, it has to be an individual choice on Aileen's part if she wants to continue to get a move on, or indeed to move on with her career independently of her colleagues. She may have to leave her workmates behind as she progresses on her chosen path, and that outcome has to be heard in its widest context: only Aileen can decide where it applies.

Becoming an individual is a lonely and courageous path, and not everyone chooses it. But it is our hero's journey in life; it is the vocation our unconscious ordains for us. An individual – distinguished from others by our own qualities – is what we are meant to become. Regretfully, in Aileen's case, it may entail having to leave others behind if the pace of her Persona is different to theirs.

Bridget's dream of her front teeth falling out

◆ ✧ ◆ ✧ ◆

I dreamed that my front teeth fell out. I was holding my hand under my chin and spitting them out. – Bridget

◆ ✧ ◆ ✧ ◆

Losing our teeth is an experience that all of us have had. We lose our milk teeth as children, spitting them out. And there are photographs in most households of grinning children with toothy gaps in their mouths! This marks a stage in our growth towards adulthood. What's unusual in this dream is that Bridget's front teeth fall out when she's an adult, and this indicates that there's something wrong. So while this is a Persona dream to do with appearances, it's also a warning dream.

Bridget isn't spitting these teeth directly onto the ground, rather, she's catching them in the hand under her chin, which suggests she's looking at what she's doing, and recognising that her teeth have value and importance.

The obvious question to ask is whether Bridget has a health problem to do with her teeth, and whether they are in need of attention. If that isn't the case, then Bridget's unconscious is staging this dream to bring something else to her attention.

To lose our front teeth strikes a blow at our outward appearance, our Persona that we present to the public. It interferes with our smile and makes us self-conscious. It's normally something that we would try to disguise, so could Bridget be concealing something, and from whom? If so, her unconscious isn't happy with keeping secrets, and is telling her they need to be spit out.

We use our teeth to ingest food, and metaphorically if we chew on something and it damages our teeth, it means that we're not able to take it in. Perhaps there's a reality facing Bridget that she's unable to deal with, to such an extent that her teeth fall out in her attempt to get to grips with it. There are many phrases referring to teeth in the language that maybe could shed light on Bridget's difficulty: a kick in the teeth, to fling in a person's teeth, as scarce as hen's teeth, fed up to the teeth, in the teeth of, to make a person's teeth water, set your teeth on edge, armed to the teeth, and so on. Do any of them apply?

We all remember that as children our teeth used to fall out as we got older. So this dream can be understood as a metaphor for facing the challenges of ageing, which again links in with the experience we had as children marking that transition from milk teeth to adult teeth, with the risk of regressing back to childhood for an adult. A maturing transition is taking place in Bridget's life to which she is not paying sufficient attention or getting to grips with, and the dream is alerting her to this.

Finally, we bring dental problems to the attention of a dentist: in other words, we ask for outside help with our teeth. I mentioned that this is a warning dream, and since it's couched in terms of teeth falling out, it suggests the need for outside, remedial help. So whatever difficulties Bridget finds herself in at the moment, it might be a good idea to talk them over with someone she trusts, so that she can avail of whatever help is on offer.

Catherine's dream of her face covered in acne

✦ ✧ ✦ ✧ ✦

I dreamt that my face was covered in acne. All
I wanted to do was cry and hide. Everyone was
looking at me and my face felt hard and then I
got sick. When I woke up I went to the mirror
and my face was fine, but it really scared me.
– Catherine

✦ ✧ ✦ ✧ ✦

*T*he drama of this Persona dream shows that Catherine feels
she daren't show her face. The bottom line in her dream
seems to be that she's afraid of other people's judgement; that
they would ridicule her, in this instance, because her face is
covered in acne. Catherine's reaction to this Persona problem is,
as she says, to 'cry and hide'. When she woke up from the dream
and looked in the mirror, her face was fine, 'but it really scared
me', she says. And so it should.

The dream draws Catherine's attention to the fact that she is
giving such a top priority to her feelings of insecurity over acne
that all she wants to do is 'cry and hide'. This childish attitude

needs to change. The dream doesn't show her as paraplegic, or suffering from cancer or motor neurone disease; in the dream she has a bad case of acne, which is often curable. So the dream is warning Catherine that she needs to present a harder face to the world, and devote some time to freeing herself from what others might think of her. Indeed, the dream actually emphasises through her awakening and going to the mirror that her face was fine, so the energy to achieve this change is already available to her.

Catherine needs to start believing in herself. What's required here is some self-affirmation: self-affirmation in spite of doubt, self-affirmation in spite of opposition, self-affirmation in spite of jealousy, self-affirmation in spite of fear. She should just be herself, as she is! The dream says that there's nothing wrong with her, particularly with her appearance. So any gesture she can make – no matter how small – to change her previous way of thinking about herself and her place in the world will work towards her good.

10

The Symbolic Language of Dreams

S ymbolic language is the one language that all of us share as human beings, because it speaks of experiences that have been common to all humanity through our evolutionary history. The wisdom in symbolic language rests on the myth-making facility of the human mind.

Dreams are both figurative and phonetic, corresponding to the two hemispheres of the human brain. The word 'figurative' comes from the Latin 'figura', meaning shape. It has to do with the right side of the brain, which processes the pictorial representation that creates the image in the dream – an essentially visual presentation. It tends to be intuitive, ambiguous, humorous and, of course, emotional. It's also metaphorical, where an idea or action is transferred onto a different object or action that's analogous to it. For example, referring to a child as 'that monkey'.

The word 'phonetic' comes from the Greek verb '*phonein*', meaning to speak. It has to do with the left side of the brain, using the discursive activity of spoken sounds or speech. It is more literal, logical, precise, consistent and cold. The left hemisphere is responsible for rational, empirical thinking, as well as language. And it is metonymic in its workings, meaning it can replace the name of one thing with the attribute of something else closely associated to it, for example, using the White House to represent the presidency of the United States.

In the human brain, the left hemisphere is a relatively new addition in evolutionary terms. The left frontal cortex, which is responsible for rational thinking as well as speech, exercises a degree of control over the right hemisphere, which is emotional and has to do with feeding, fighting, fleeing and fornication. This dominant forebrain has been characterised as Promethian, relating to the bringer of light and consciousness, while the more ancient part of the brain has been denigrated as Epimethian, relating to the bearer of darkness and unconsciousness. Since it doesn't possess the gift of speech, the right hemisphere, containing the limbic affectional system, has to phrase its communications from the unconscious in symbols, which both parts of the brain can understand. The conscious forebrain collaborates in this with speech as well as with a gift for telling stories, transforming these symbolic messages into narrative form. The result is the symbolic language of dreams, which combines the figurative with the phonetic. So the meaning of our dreams is expressed in a pictorial language that we can construe only when its images are put into words – especially our own words, the words that we use every day.

Incubation is the religious practice of sleeping in a sacred space or consecrated ground in order to have a divinely inspired dream. In ancient Greece, when a patient incubated a dream in temples sacred to the god of medicine, Asclepius, it required no interpretation because the dream experience was itself the instrument of healing that provided the cure. The vast majority of our dreams are never interpreted, but they serve their purpose because we experience the psychic reality of the dream while we're asleep. In our dreams, we live out the total spectrum of our being, and fulfil all of our potential. The unconscious and consciousness are at one in the attainment of this goal. Dream amnesia seems to be built into the system lest we behave as if the dreams were real, which would defeat this creative, healing purpose.

In interpreting a dream, we enter the atmosphere of the dream to establish its mood, as well as the detail of its images and symbols, in such a way as to amplify the experience of the dream itself. Then its impact on our consciousness is enhanced. And the remarkable feature of the dream's content lies in our ability to express in symbolic or metaphorical terms the connection with a current problem or aspect of our past experience that relates to the problem, concentrating primarily on the aspects that the psyche wants us to deal with.

Dreams are a form of symbolic communication whose meaning is governed by context. As we explore the contextual web through which the dream images are interconnected, their overall significance emerges as a gradual revelation, like developing a photographic film chemically. It's not a question of getting the right interpretation, but of allowing the dream to speak for itself and express all of its meanings, which can never be exhausted.

Declan's dream of carrying loads of things from one room to another

✦ ✧ ✦ ✧ ✦

I always dream that I had to carry loads of things from one room to another and my hands feel swollen when doing so. Even when I wake up they feel the same. Why do I keep having this dream? – Declan

✦ ✧ ✦ ✧ ✦

*D*reams are a metaphor for something that's going on in real life. So what can we tell from Declan's dream? He says, 'I always dream that I had to carry loads of things ... and my hands feel swollen when doing so.' Declan is carrying too much baggage, so much so that his hands feel swollen under the weight of it all. In addition, he says, 'I always dream', meaning that this is a recurring dream. So to answer Declan's question of why he keeps having this dream, it's repeating because it is asking him to pay attention to this situation he finds himself in, and to do something about being overloaded.

Declan doesn't say whether the dream refers to having too much work on his plate, or whether the 'loads of things' he talks about are a representation of his psychological baggage, or maybe even physical weight that he's carrying. In any case, he has to shed these because they're just too heavy.

Maybe Declan should give some consideration to talking to someone he trusts about the pressure he's under. The dream brings to his attention that the load is having a physical effect: as Declan says, 'my hands feel swollen ... Even when I wake up they feel the same.' This dream is a warning that a solution has to be found for the difficulty dramatised here if Declan is to remain physically healthy. Swelling in part of the body is a condition called 'oedema', and it is a subject that Declan might consider discussing with his doctor at his next check-up if they continue to feel the same, to make sure that there's no underlying medical problem.

Emmett's dream of holding the baby

✦ ✧ ✦ ✧ ✦

I had a dream that I was in a shopping centre and a woman asked whether I would mind holding her baby while she went to the bathroom. I said fine. She didn't come back. I checked the toilet but she was gone. The panic was extreme. – Emmett

✦ ✧ ✦ ✧ ✦

*T*he dream shows that Emmett is left holding the baby! He's literally responsible for another human being, who's helpless and cannot look after itself. And he was tricked into doing this. It leaves him with a feeling of extreme panic. So where in Emmett's life has a woman tricked him into a role of responsibility, but for something that's not his personal responsibility? Even in the drama of the dream, while there's momentary panic, it's to be expected that Emmett will eventually ring the Gardaí and hand the baby over to the authorities, who will relieve him of that huge responsibility, which doesn't belong to him. After all, it's 'her baby'.

The dream paints this picture in dramatic form to get Emmett's attention that he is being over-responsible, that he has been left holding a baby for someone else. He needs to confront this situation head on. The dream infers that Emmett needs to tell the authorities – someone independent from outside the situation in which he finds himself – that he isn't going to continue to do this, and in that way be relieved of someone else's responsibility.

The Trickster motif in this dream is clear in that Emmett has been tricked into helplessly holding the baby. But the dream needs the further step of Emmett being tricked into the mature response of refusing to comply, and dealing responsibly with what has been presented in the drama of his dream.

Frank's dream of swimming in a cube

✦ ✧ ✦ ✧ ✦

I dreamt that I was swimming in a cube almost full of water. It was spinning, and I had to keep swimming to the top of the cube as it spun. The cube was in space, and I could see the earth. Any idea what it's about? – Frank

✦ ✧ ✦ ✧ ✦

There's an alarming quality to the metaphor of this dream. Frank says he's swimming in a cube almost full of water, and that he had to keep swimming to the top of the cube, presumably to keep his head above water because otherwise he would drown. So the dream shows that Frank is in a precarious situation, fighting for his life. Not only that, but the cube was spinning, so Frank is being spun around. From his perspective inside the cube, everything is spinning out of control.

According to the dream, the cube was in space and Frank could see the earth. So Frank is absolutely on his own, out in the cold, abandoned in outer space and spinning out of control. Space is an alien environment in which human beings can't survive, unless they are astronauts with a massive support team on earth backing them up. So Frank asks, 'Any ideas what it's about?'

The dream paints Frank a picture of the isolated nature of his situation, which his psyche considers to be very dangerous indeed for him. It's asking him to pay attention to what's happening, and to get out of the spinning situation he is in right now before he drowns. If he doesn't do anything, he will inevitably use up his resources, and won't be able to continue to keep his head above water.

So Frank needs to heed the stark warning of the dream. His psyche has his best interests at heart, and if he follows the direction plotted by his inner Self – if he follows what's good for him – life will turn out to be a success, rather than the opposite, which is potentiality threatened in his dream.

Tessa's dream of driving her car

✦ ✧ ✦ ✧ ✦

I keep dreaming I'm driving my car. It's always around my neighbourhood area. I feel stressed in the dream. I work with computers, so don't drive a lot during the day. – Tessa

✦ ✧ ✦ ✧ ✦

There are positives and negatives in this dream. The positives are that Tessa is driving her car: she's in the driving seat, controlling what's going on. And she's driving around her neighbourhood area, so she's familiar with the location and presumably she knows the neighbours and also how the road system in her area works. All good so far.

Then come the negatives: Tessa says that she 'feels stressed in the dream'. In other words, she has some anxiety, but she doesn't say what that anxiety is. However, the next statement is 'I work with computers'. So could that be the source of the anxiety and stress? The full sentence is: 'I work with computers, so don't drive a lot during the day.' This implies that to drive her car during working hours is unusual, or to put it another way, to be in charge of her car, and to be in the driving seat during working hours, is unusual. The car is a metaphor for horsepower, energy and freedom – for being able to move about, being in control, maybe even self-esteem, and so on. And Tessa also says, 'I don't drive a lot during the day', which tells us that her drive is lowered during the day!

So we need to join the two sections together – the positive and negative. When Tessa is in a familiar situation and in the driving seat, she feels stressed, and at face value the stress arises 'around my neighbourhood area'. The original meaning of the word 'neighbourhood' referred to friendly relations between neighbours. Are the friendly relationships in her home area still in place, and if not, is that breakdown the source of Tessa's stress? She adds, 'I work with computers'. So a question is: does she have too much responsibility at work; is that the pressure point? The word 'stress' means pressure or coercion, in the sense of being confined or controlled, so that, too, is a possibility.

I think the dream points out to Tessa that she has no need to be stressed in familiar situations when she's in the driving seat. It tells her that she is well able for the challenge – it's as easy as driving her car around her neighbourhood area. And since she doesn't drive a lot during the day, the drama of the dream compensates for her being confined and controlled working with computers by staging an escape and going for a drive. Since Tessa keeps dreaming this type of dream, she needs to take a serious look at her work situation, and decide how she can improve the stresses involved and handle them differently. Once these solutions are implemented, then this type of dream will stop.

Garvan's dream of being on top of a massive crane

✦ ✧ ✦ ✧ ✦

I had a dream that I was on top of a massive unstable crane. It started spinning out of control and flipping and I almost fell off. I was petrified. There were two strangers up there with me. I was then taken onto a fishing boat by its skipper, which was also scary. – Garvan

✦ ✧ ✦ ✧ ✦

Garvan is in a very dangerous situation, which is out of the ordinary. He says he is 'on top of a massive unstable crane', which 'started spinning out of control and flipping, and I almost fell off'. Garvan is not grounded – he's literally flying far too high. Nobody should be on top of a crane in the first place, if they don't know how to handle it.

The important phrase here is 'spinning out of control'. Whatever situation Garvan is in in real life, it's registering in his psyche as being 'out of control' and 'spinning'. Garvan's reaction is to say, 'I was petrified.' The origin of the word 'petrify' comes from the Latin and Greek word '*petra*', meaning rock.

So 'petrificare' means to make or become stone. It was the Irish writer Oliver Goldsmith who first used the word in its figurative sense, which is to change as if to stone, to benumb or to paralyse with fear and horror. And this is what Garvan is saying happens to him in his dream: he's paralysed with fear and horror.

He concludes, 'I was then taken onto a fishing boat by its skipper, which was also scary.' The good thing about this conclusion in the dream is that going on a fishing boat is a normal occurrence, even though it might be scary for someone who hasn't done it before. The other important point to bear in mind is that the skipper is there so the boat is under the control of someone who knows what he's doing. So Garvan is now safe from the elements.

If we take both parts of the dream together – being on top of a crane out of control and being on a fishing boat under the control of its skipper – we can see that the movement in Garvan's dream is from being 'petrified' with fear to being 'scary'. This shows that Garvan has the resources within to be captain of his own ship, and to handle what is happening in his life. He can bring down whatever is happening to manageable proportions and deal with it. And because the dream is screaming at Garvan in nightmare form, he really must take steps to let his inner skipper take charge, and deal immediately with the dangerous circumstance in which he's spinning out of control and heading for a fall.

Ian's dream of being able to fly

✦ ✧ ✦ ✧ ✦

*I dream a lot that if I run fast and flap my arms
I take off and can fly up high over everything.
I've had this dream for years. – Ian*

✦ ✧ ✦ ✧ ✦

This is a dream of the impossible, because human beings can't fly! Although, to be fair to Ian, our shoulder blades resemble the rudimentary remains of wings. Certainly, our ape cousins 'fly' about from branch to branch in the jungle, so to succeed at 'flying' today would be a throwback to an earlier form of being: we'd have to regress to being more primitive.

Ian's wish as shown in his dream is to be able to 'fly up high over everything'. So what is the metaphor that constantly runs through Ian's head when he's sleeping? He wants to be above the fray, to get away from it all, to escape, to take flight, or to 'run fast', as he says. This means he wants to run away, instead of being humble and accepting his limitations and getting down and dirty on the ground. And the dream constantly brings this to Ian's attention, as he says, 'I've had this dream for years.'

Dreams work to restore our psychic balance. And this recurring dream of flying also suggests that Ian is trying to get above himself through having unrealistic ideas or too high an opinion of himself, or making grandiose plans out of all proportion to his actual abilities. So Ian needs to face up to reality and accept the limits we all live with. Ian might as well make the best of it, remain firmly grounded, and deal with what is presented to him. As adults, we have the power to change things if we don't like them, so he should confront whatever needs to be changed in his life, and put a plan in place. That's how Ian will really soar!

Jeremiah's dream of a storm hitting the house

✦ ✧ ✦ ✧ ✦

I dream a lot that I'm asleep in bed and a storm hits the house. It blows in the windows, goes right through the room and is really violent. Even though this storm is around the bed, I feel calm. – Jeremiah

✦ ✧ ✦ ✧ ✦

J eremiah says that even though this storm is really violent, he feels calm. And on the face of it, remaining calm in the face of violence seems to be a good attitude to have. But let's look at this dream more closely.

Jeremiah says he is asleep and a storm hits the house. It blows in the windows, goes right through the room and is really violent. I think he is having this dream in order to wake up to a very dangerous and life-threatening situation. I would respectfully suggest that being asleep and feeling calm in the face of a storm of such violence that the windows are blown in is inappropriate: Jeremiah needs to take action.

What is this violent storm that he dreams about a lot? Could it be anger or tension, and where is it coming from? Jeremiah says that the storm is around the bed, so does it refer to sex? Whatever it is, the problem needs to be addressed urgently if he is dreaming about it 'a lot'. So a little less calmness and more action is required to make where he lives – the house, or the reality in which he lives, or his habitual way of approaching matters – a safer place.

While a wind can be violent and destructive, in mythological terms, it's life-giving, blowing away the old and allowing something new to emerge. For example, the Hebrew word 'ruach' refers to wind or spirit, and it equates with divine inspiration and a divine voice. So this visitation in Jeremiah's dreams presages something new about to happen. The action he takes to protect himself from violence should incorporate the potential for change in some way. He needs to try out new ways of dealing with life. He can only then really afford to be calm, having taken all necessary measures to protect himself from such violence, enabling him to consciously live his life creatively inspired by the winds blowing in from his unconscious.

Luke's dream of his eighth birthday

✦ ✧ ✦ ✧ ✦

I dreamt that it was my eighth birthday. Everything in the dream was tiny – us, the house we were in, the cake, everything. There was a radio on, which kept repeating 'sun shines slowly' over and over and over. When I woke I could still hear it ringing in my head. – Luke

✦ ✧ ✦ ✧ ✦

Since the opening sentence of Luke's dream is very specific, we have to ask the question, what happened on Luke's eighth birthday? What are his memories of that day: where was he; what class was he in; what was going on in the house at the time? Was there in fact a birthday party, and if there was, who was at it?

Luke says, 'Everything in the dream was tiny – us, the house we were in, the cake, everything.' If he was eight years old, everything around him would have seemed big since he was physically so small. So in the dream he is looking back at this moment from the perspective of an adult, where things are much smaller than he remembers.

A disembodied voice comes from the radio, which repeats the phrase 'sun shines slowly', as Luke says, 'over and over and over'. This wakes him up, so we know this particular phrase is very important. What is obvious is the alliteration of the letter 's': 'sun shines slowly'. To pronounce the 's', we have to exhale. I'd also like to ask Luke what the phrase means to him. What does he hear in the phrase 'sun shines slowly' as he exhales and stops holding his breath and relaxes?

The phrase has to do with time. When we're children, we live in an eternal present, free from responsibilities. The sun shines slowly all day long, and the world exists for us eternally without being obscured by the regrets of the past or worries for the future.

When Luke awoke, he could still hear the phrase ringing in his head, repeating. So the dream has reached out into his waking life, and urges him to put into practice the mindfulness lesson of 'sun shines slowly'. In Buddhism, while mindfulness comes from the Nepali term *sati*, which refers to memory, it also refers to a term continually repeated in Buddhist practice: 'mindful and thoughtful'. Presence of mind would be a useful analogy. It is repeated for Luke in the phrase 'sun shines slowly', so that he can fully inhabit the present – be present to the present – which is the essential experience of his life.

I think the dream is a compensation for something happening in Luke's adult world today. The dream reminds Luke of a happy time, his eighth birthday, when situations were tiny and not overwhelming, when the sun shone slowly all the day long and there was no time pressure. The dream brings this to Luke's attention because it wants him to incorporate that ease and carefree happiness into his present way of life, so that he can achieve a better work/life balance, which in today's world is most likely skewed in favour of work. Luke's eighth birthday was also a simple time of innocent happiness – he mentions 'the cake'!

Luke should embrace playtime as it is the most creative thing we can do. The artist Pablo Picasso said: 'It took me four years to paint like Raphael, but a lifetime to paint like a child.' Luke must bring back the joy and wonder of that eight-year-old inside him, and he will enrich his life in ways he can only dream of!

Endnote

*I*f you've enjoyed reading this book, please tell others about it, and recommend *Michael Murphy's Book of Dreams* to your friends.

I hope the way that the various dreams have been analysed has shown you how to work with your own dreams. Regrettably I'm not in a position to engage in personal correspondence, but if you have any comments or insights about this book that you want to share, you can email me: info@michaelmurphyauthor. com.

For your added enjoyment, the website gives further background information on the book. It also gives information about the various book signings and talks around the country, where I look forward to having an opportunity to meet you, and maybe discussing in person a dream that may be troubling you. There's also a section on the website dealing with my other publications.

Thank you for taking the time to read my book of dreams. I'd like also to offer my personal thanks to everyone who submitted their dreams anonymously for analysis.

Go dté tu slán!

Michael Murphy

www.michaelmurphyauthor.com

www.psychologicaltherapyservices.com

Acknowledgements

*T*hank you Sarah Liddy for commissioning this book, and to Catherine Gough and the editorial team at Gill Books, in particular my copy-editor, Ellen Christie. A big thank you is also due to Teresa Daly and Gill's marketing team, and it's great to work again with Paul Nielan in the sales department!

I'm indebted to my own team of devoted friends: my literary agent and publicist, Fiona Coffey, my researcher and tour manager, Margaret Martin, and my co-presenter on the road, Ciana Campbell. Thank you for the fun and for clearing the way.

Kevin Cassidy and Paul Power of the Park Studio give unstinting technical support, and Dave Douglas and Sharon Murray at Ebow keep my website up to date. For them, nothing is too much trouble.

The radio producer Therese Kelly first issued the invitation to analyse people's dreams on the 2FM *Chris and Ciara Show*, and she granted permission to include some of them here. Marie Toft, television producer on the afternoon *Today Show*, honed the helpful responses required in live broadcasting. To all the production teams in Dublin and Cork, and in particular to Chris and Ciara, Maura and Daithí, I extend my gratitude for their kindness.

I wish to acknowledge the honour Dr Patrick Randall, Ireland's foremost forensic psychologist, has accorded this book by contributing the foreword. I feel privileged availing of his erudition and endorsement.

Mi amigo argentino en españa, José Luis Veiga, took the cover photograph. And profound gratitude is also due to my honorary family member in Spain, Anna Timmermann (one of the Murphys of Copenhagen!) for her unconditional support.

My friend Vickie Maye, features editor of the *Irish Examiner,* gives me ongoing encouragment via emails at dawn when both of us are at our desks.

Finally, my partner, Terry, allows me the time to write. He is my own Wise Old Man, on whom I depend.

All of these people, who are so publicly professional, offer me personal support for which I'm profoundly grateful.

Rath Dé oraibh uilig.

Also by the Author

Prose
At Five in the Afternoon
The House of Pure Being
Lemons and the Waning Moon (forthcoming)

Poetry
The Republic of Love
A Chaplet of Roses